I0623014

PROTEIN

pil
Publications International, Ltd.

Louis Weber, CEO
Publications International, Ltd.
5250 Old Orchard Road, Suite 500
Skokie, IL 60077

Pictured on the front cover: Simple Sushi Poke Bowls (page 146).

Pictured on the back cover *(left to right):* Smoked Salmon Omelet *(page 22)* and Lentil Ragù *(page 170)*.

ISBN: 979-8-89746-146-2

Manufactured in China.

8 7 6 5 4 3 2 1

Microwave Cooking: Microwave ovens vary in wattage. Use the cooking times as guidelines and check for doneness before adding more time.

Note: This publication is only intended to provide general information. The information is specifically not intended to be a substitute for medical diagnosis or treatment by your physician or other health care professional. You should always consult your own physician` or other health care professionals about any medical questions, diagnosis, or treatment. (Products vary among manufacturers. Please check labels carefully to confirm nutritional values.)

The information obtained by you from this book should not be relied upon for any personal, nutritional, or medical decision. You should consult an appropriate professional for specific advice tailored to your specific situation. PIL makes no representations or warranties, express or implied, with respect to your use of this information.

In no event shall PIL, its affiliates or advertisers be liable for any direct, indirect, punitive, incidental, special, or consequential damages, or any damages whatsoever including, without limitation, damages for personal injury, death, damage to property, or loss of profits, arising out of or in any way connected with the use of any of the above-referenced information or otherwise arising out of the use of this book.

Nutritional Analysis: Every effort has been made to check the accuracy of the nutritional information that appears with each recipe. However, because numerous variables account for a wide range of values for certain foods, nutritive analyses in this book should be considered approximate.

WARNING: Food preparation, baking and cooking involve inherent dangers: misuse of electric products, sharp electric tools, boiling water, hot stoves, allergic reactions, foodborne illnesses and the like, pose numerous potential risks. Publications International, Ltd. (PIL) assumes no responsibility or liability for any damages you may experience as a result of following recipes, instructions, tips or advice in this publication.

While we hope this publication helps you find new ways to eat delicious foods, you may not always achieve the results desired due to variations in ingredients, cooking temperatures, typos, errors, omissions or individual cooking abilities.

CONTENTS

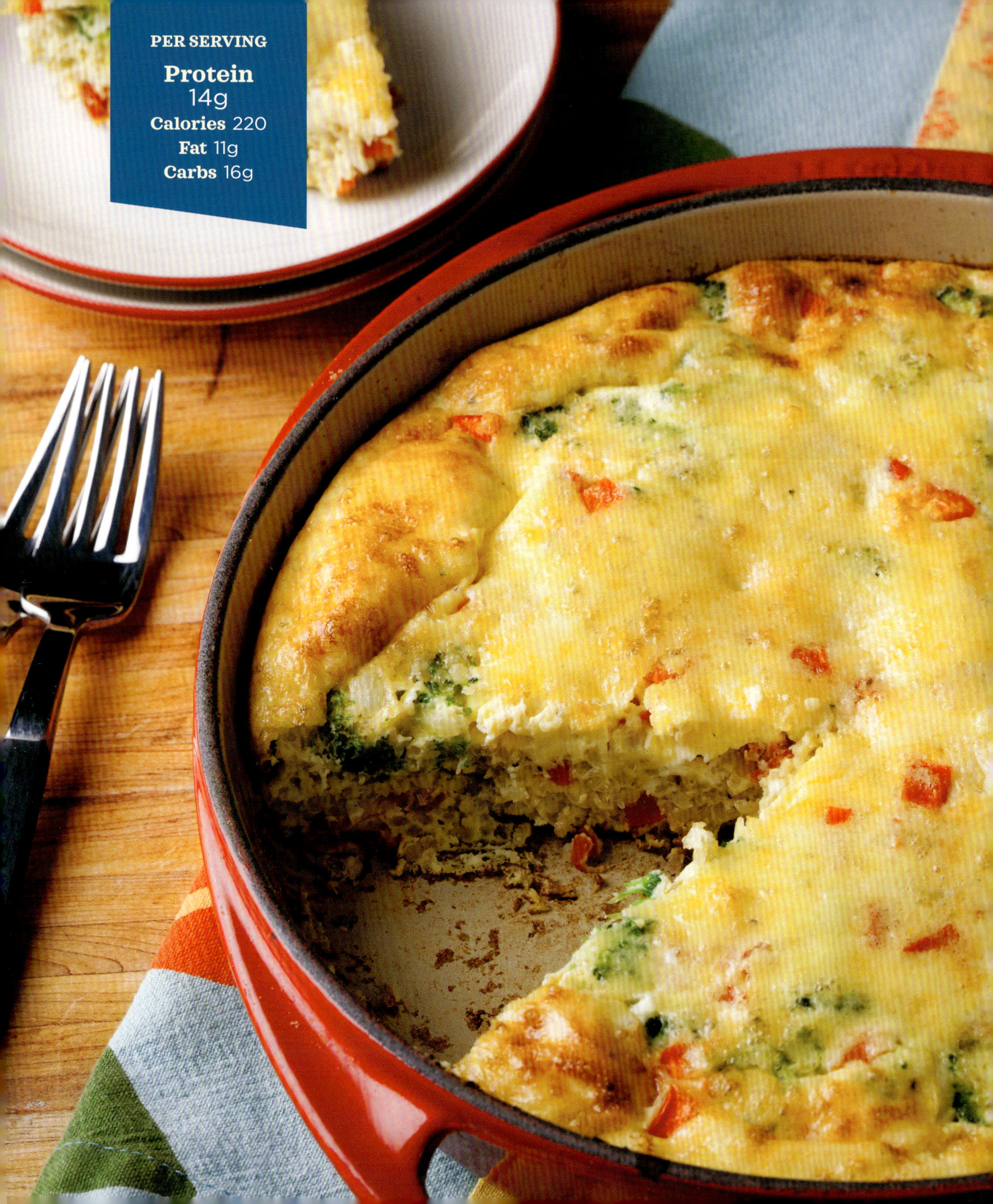
PER SERVING
Protein
14g
Calories 220
Fat 11g
Carbs 16g

BREAKFAST

Vegetable Quinoa Frittata

MAKES 6 SERVINGS

- **1 tablespoon olive oil**
- **1 cup chopped onion**
- **1 cup small broccoli florets**
- **¾ cup finely chopped red bell pepper**
- **2 cloves garlic, minced**
- **1¼ teaspoons coarse salt**
- **Black pepper**
- **1½ cups cooked quinoa (see Tip)**
- **¼ cup sun-dried tomatoes, chopped**
- **8 eggs, lightly beaten**
- **¼ cup grated Parmesan cheese**

1. Preheat oven to 400°F.
2. Heat oil in large ovenproof skillet over medium-high heat. Add onion and broccoli; cook and stir 4 minutes, Add bell pepper; cook and stir 2 minutes. Add garlic, salt and black pepper; cook and stir 30 seconds. Stir in quinoa and sun-dried tomatoes.
3. Gently stir in eggs; cook until softly scrambled. Sprinkle with cheese.
4. Bake 7 minutes or until center is set. Let stand 5 minutes before cutting into wedges.

Tip

For 1½ cups cooked quinoa, use ½ cup uncooked (dry) quinoa.

Mediterranean Artichoke Omelet

MAKES 1 SERVING

- 2 eggs
- 1 tablespoon grated Parmesan cheese
- 2 tablespoons olive oil
- 3 canned artichokes, chopped
- 1 ounce (about 2 pieces) roasted red peppers, diced
- ½ teaspoon minced garlic
- 1 tablespoon tomato salsa

1. Beat eggs in small bowl; stir in cheese.
2. Heat oil in large skillet over medium-high heat. Add artichokes; cook and stir 3 minutes or until beginning to brown. Add roasted peppers; cook and stir 2 minutes or until liquid has evaporated. Add garlic; cook and stir 30 seconds. Remove to small plate; keep warm.
3. Add egg mixture to skillet. Lift edge of omelet with spatula to allow any uncooked portion to flow underneath. Cook 1 to 2 minutes or until omelet is almost set.
4. Spoon artichoke mixture onto half of omelet; fold omelet over filling. Cook 2 minutes or until set. Serve with salsa.

Note

Raw eggs will turn green if combined with raw artichokes because of a chemical reaction between the two foods. Cooking the artichokes separately prevents this from happening.

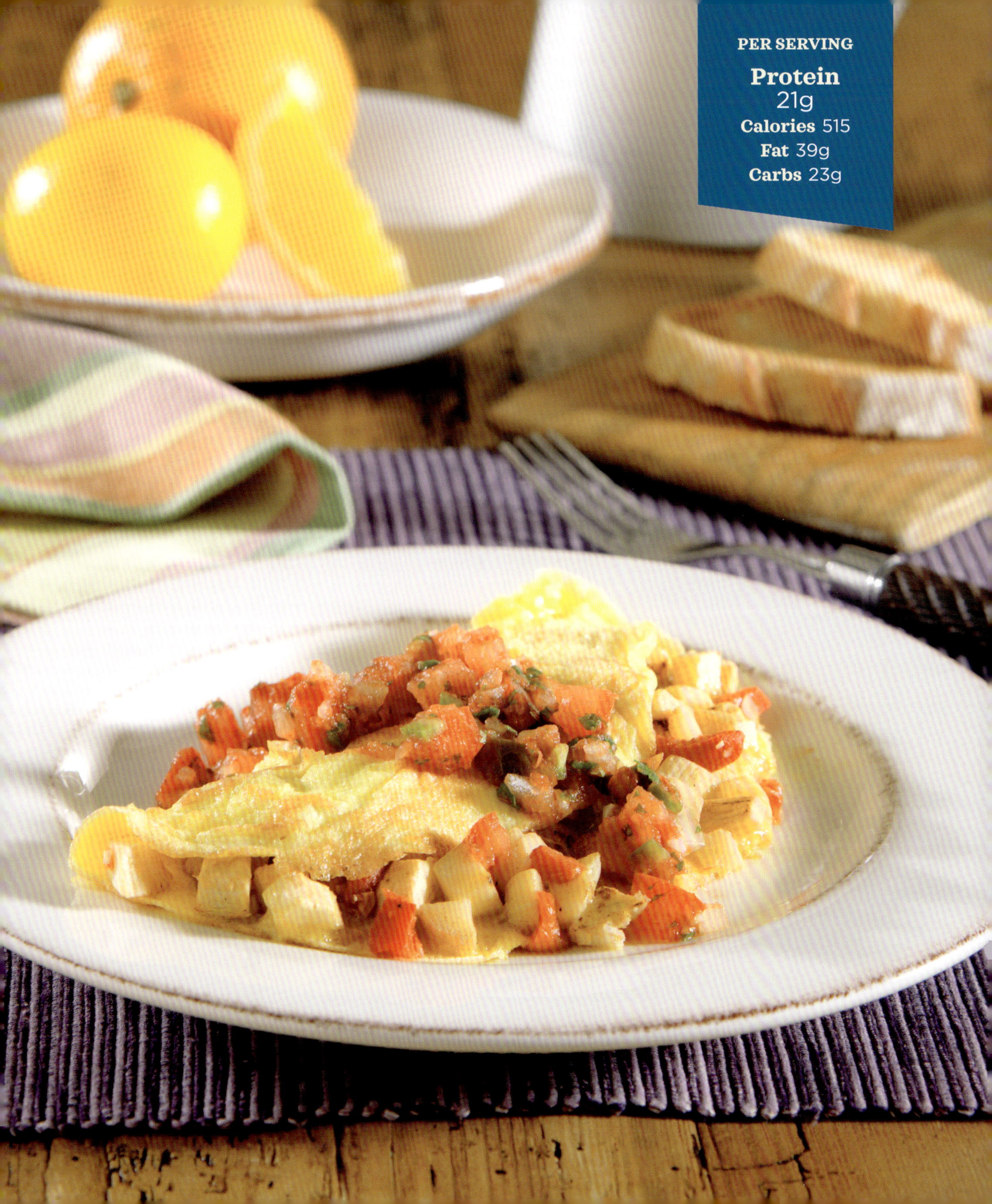

PER SERVING

Protein 21g

Calories 515

Fat 39g

Carbs 23g

PER SERVING
Protein
10g
Calories 210
Fat 4g
Carbs 36g

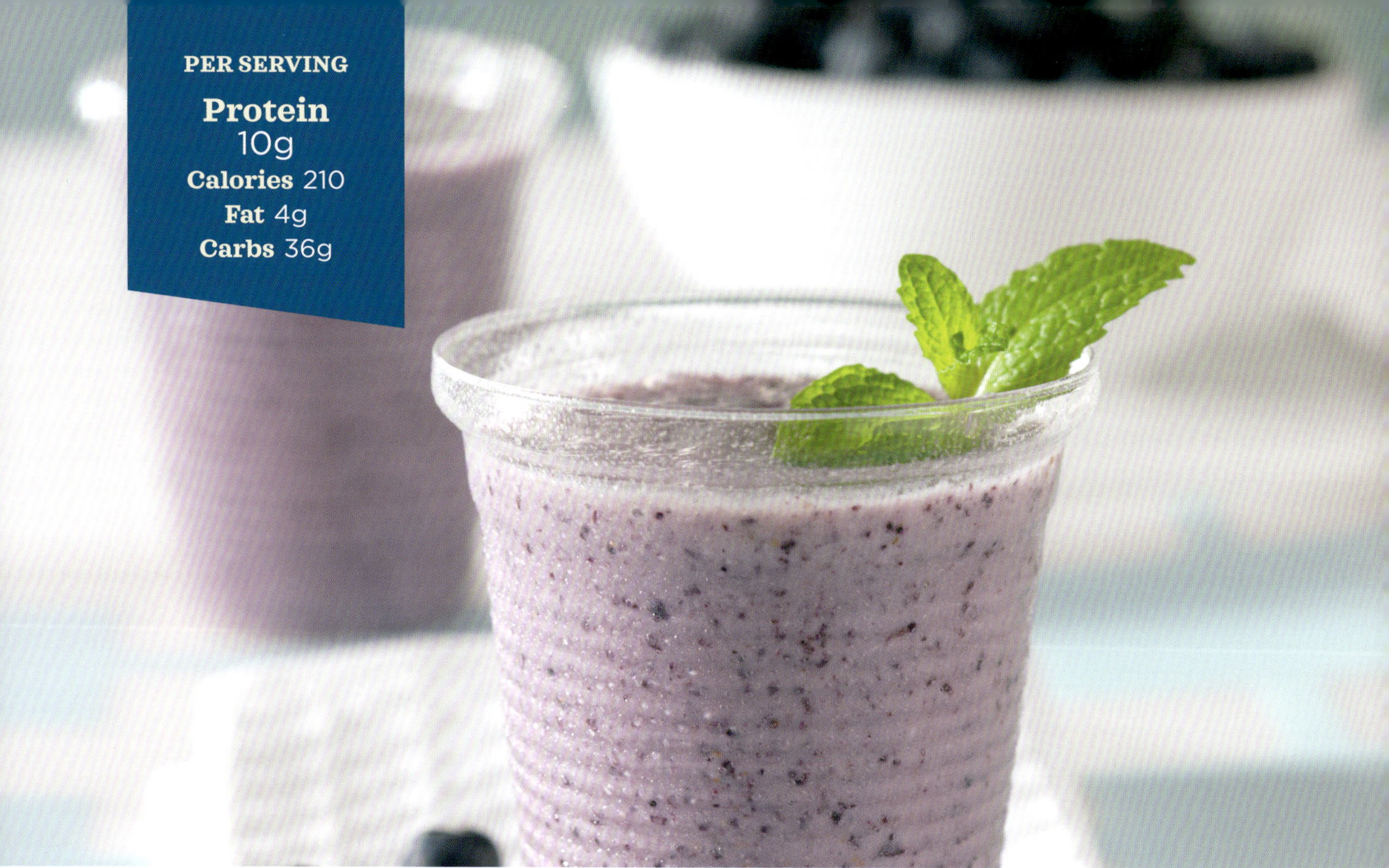

Blueberry Banana Oatmeal Smoothie

MAKES 2 SERVINGS

- **1 cup reduced-fat (2%) milk**
- **1 small ripe banana**
- **½ cup frozen blueberries**
- **½ cup plain nonfat yogurt**
- **¼ cup quick oats**
- **Fresh mint sprigs (optional)**

Combine milk, banana and blueberries in blender; blend until smooth. Add yogurt and oats; blend until smooth. Garnish with mint.

PER SERVING
Protein
19g
Calories 340
Fat 4g
Carbs 60g

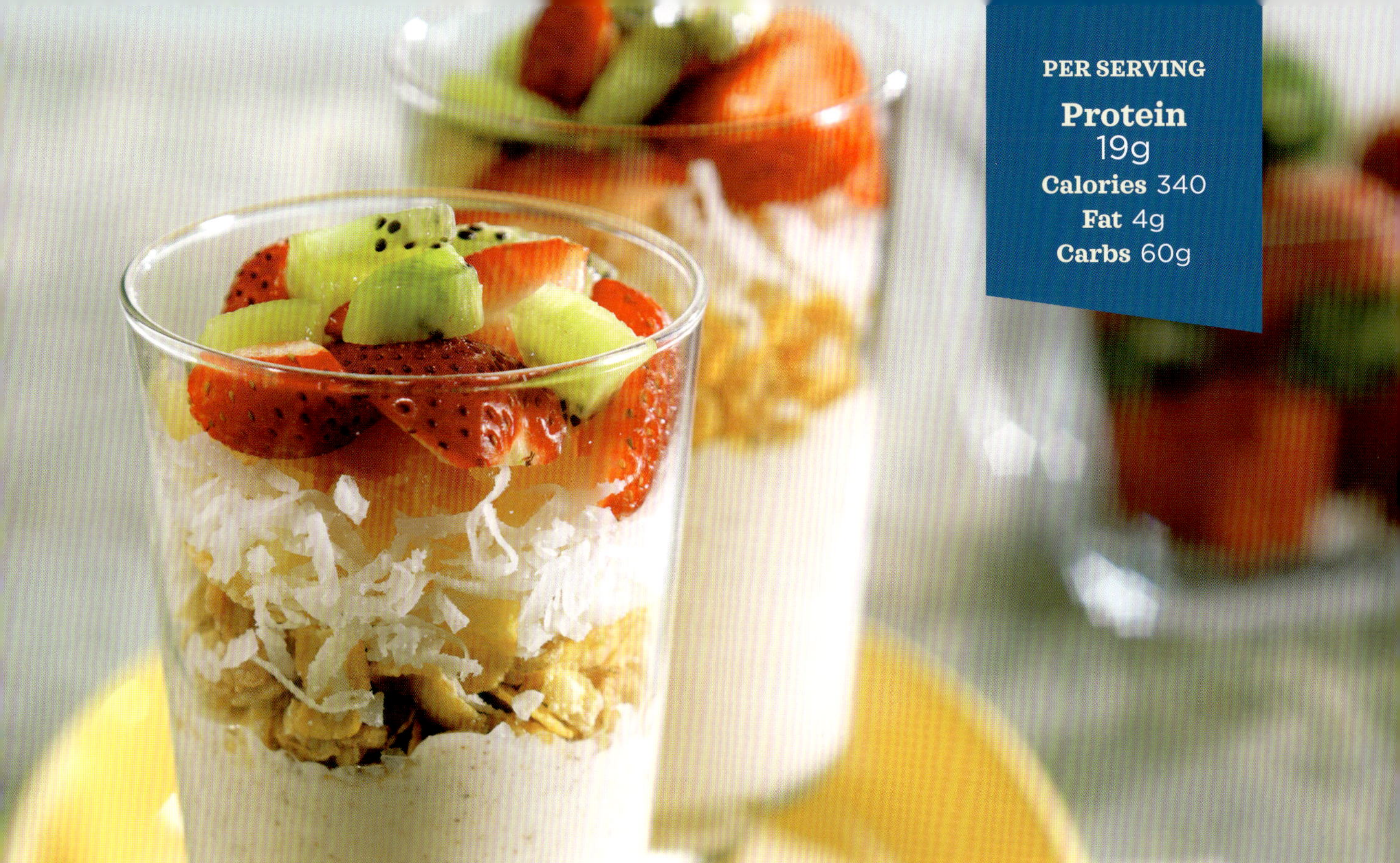

Tropical Fruit Breakfast Parfaits

MAKES 4 SERVINGS

- 1½ cups vanilla nonfat Greek yogurt
- 1 banana, mashed
- 2 tablespoons maple syrup or honey
- ¾ teaspoon ground cinnamon
- 1 cup honey-sweetened oat flakes cereal
- ½ cup flaked coconut
- 1 can (8 ounces) crushed pineapple in juice, drained
- 2 cups strawberries, quartered
- 1 kiwi, peeled and diced

1. Combine yogurt, banana, maple syrup and cinnamon in medium bowl; mix well.
2. Spoon about ⅓ cup yogurt mixture into each of four parfait or wine glasses; top with cereal, coconut and fruit.

Farmstand Frittata

MAKES 4 SERVINGS

- **1 medium red bell pepper, cut into thin strips, plus additional for garnish**
- **½ cup chopped onion**
- **1 cup cooked broccoli florets**
- **1 cup quartered cooked unpeeled new red potatoes**
- **1 cup liquid egg substitute**
- **6 egg whites**
- **1 tablespoon chopped fresh parsley**
- **½ teaspoon salt**
- **¼ teaspoon black pepper**
- **½ cup (2 ounces) shredded reduced-fat Cheddar cheese**

1. Spray large ovenproof skillet with nonstick cooking spray; heat over medium heat. Add bell pepper and onion; cook and stir 3 minutes or until vegetables are crisp-tender. Add broccoli and potatoes; cook and stir 1 to 2 minutes or until heated through.

2. Meanwhile, whisk egg substitute, egg whites, parsley, salt and black pepper in medium bowl until well blended.

3. Spread vegetables in even layer in skillet. Pour egg mixture over vegetables; cover and cook over medium heat 8 to 10 minutes or until almost set.

4. Meanwhile, preheat broiler. Sprinkle cheese over frittata; broil 2 to 3 minutes or until golden brown and set. Let stand 5 minutes before cutting into wedges. Garnish with additional bell pepper.

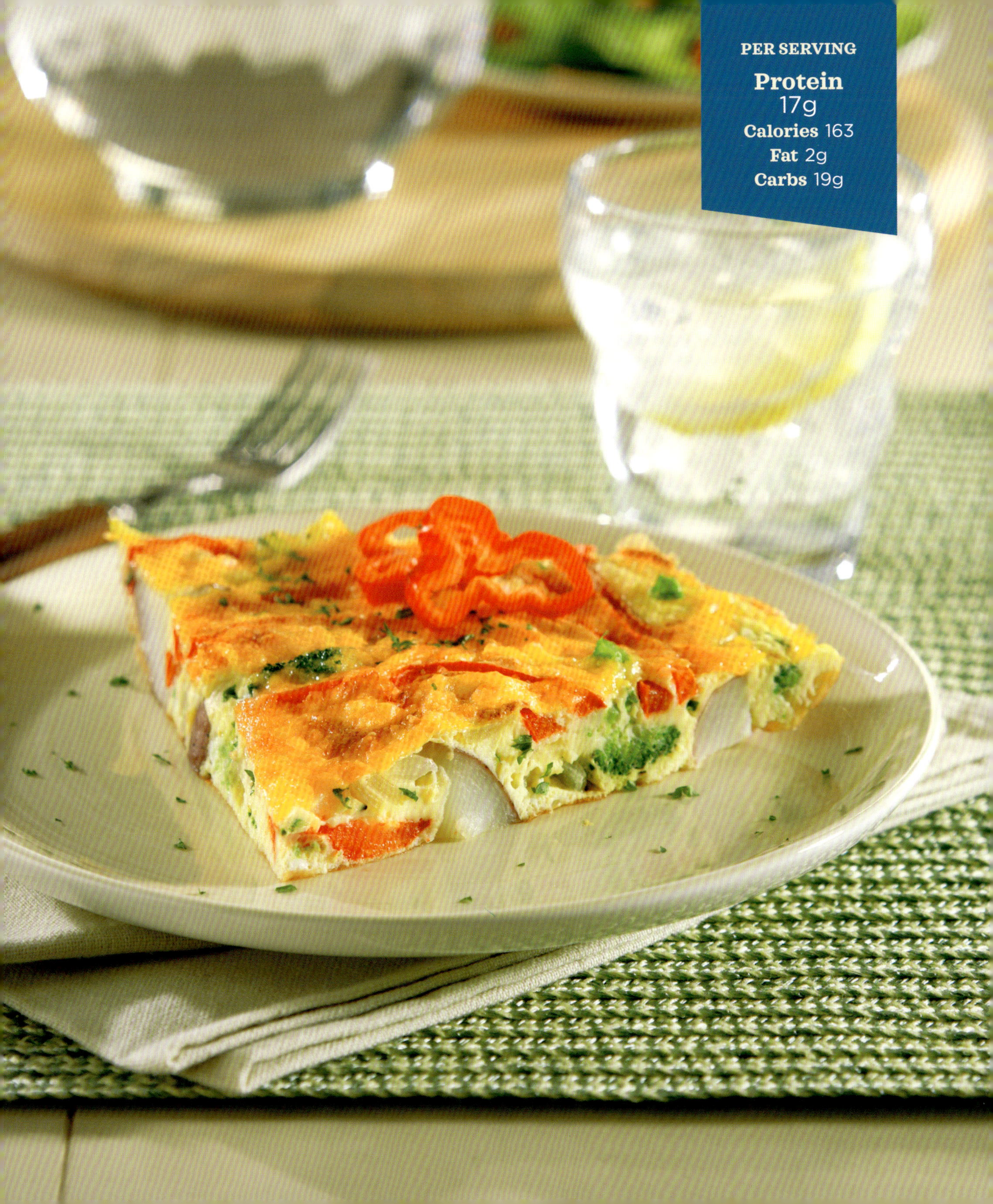
PER SERVING
Protein
17g
Calories 163
Fat 2g
Carbs 19g

PER SERVING
Protein
12g
Calories 270
Fat 8g
Carbs 36g

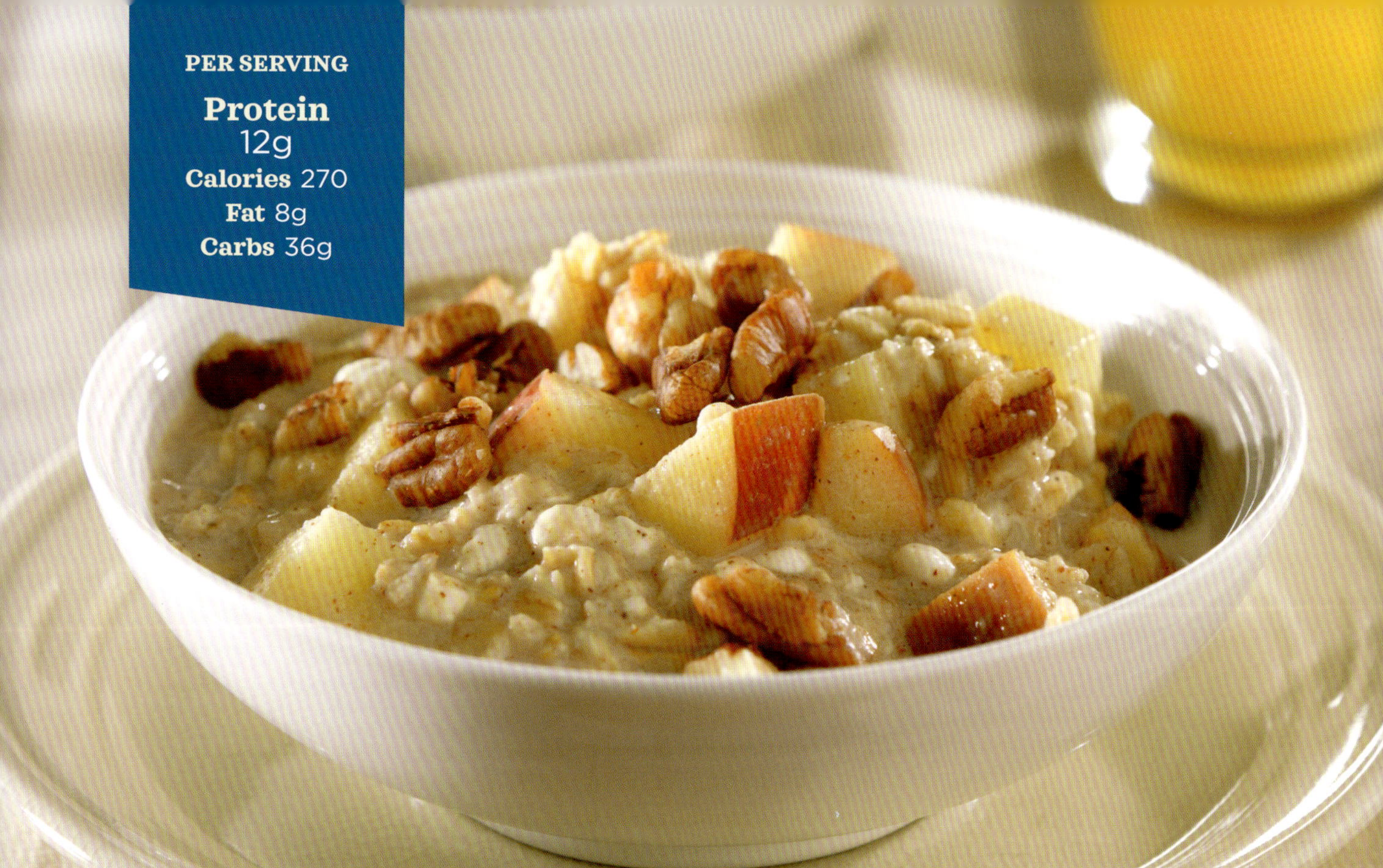

Oatmeal with Apples and Cottage Cheese

MAKES 2 SERVINGS

- ⅔ cup water
- ¼ teaspoon salt
- ½ cup old-fashioned oats
- ½ cup diced apple
- 2 tablespoons packed brown sugar
- 1 teaspoon vanilla
- ¾ teaspoon ground cinnamon
- ½ cup cottage cheese
- ¼ cup half-and-half
- 2 tablespoons chopped pecans or almonds

1. Bring water and salt to a boil in small saucepan over high heat. Stir in oats, apple, brown sugar, vanilla and cinnamon. Reduce heat to medium-low; cook and stir 3 to 5 minutes or until oats are tender and creamy.

2. Stir in cottage cheese and half-and-half; sprinkle with nuts.

PER SERVING
Protein
10g
Calories 130
Fat 9g
Carbs 3g

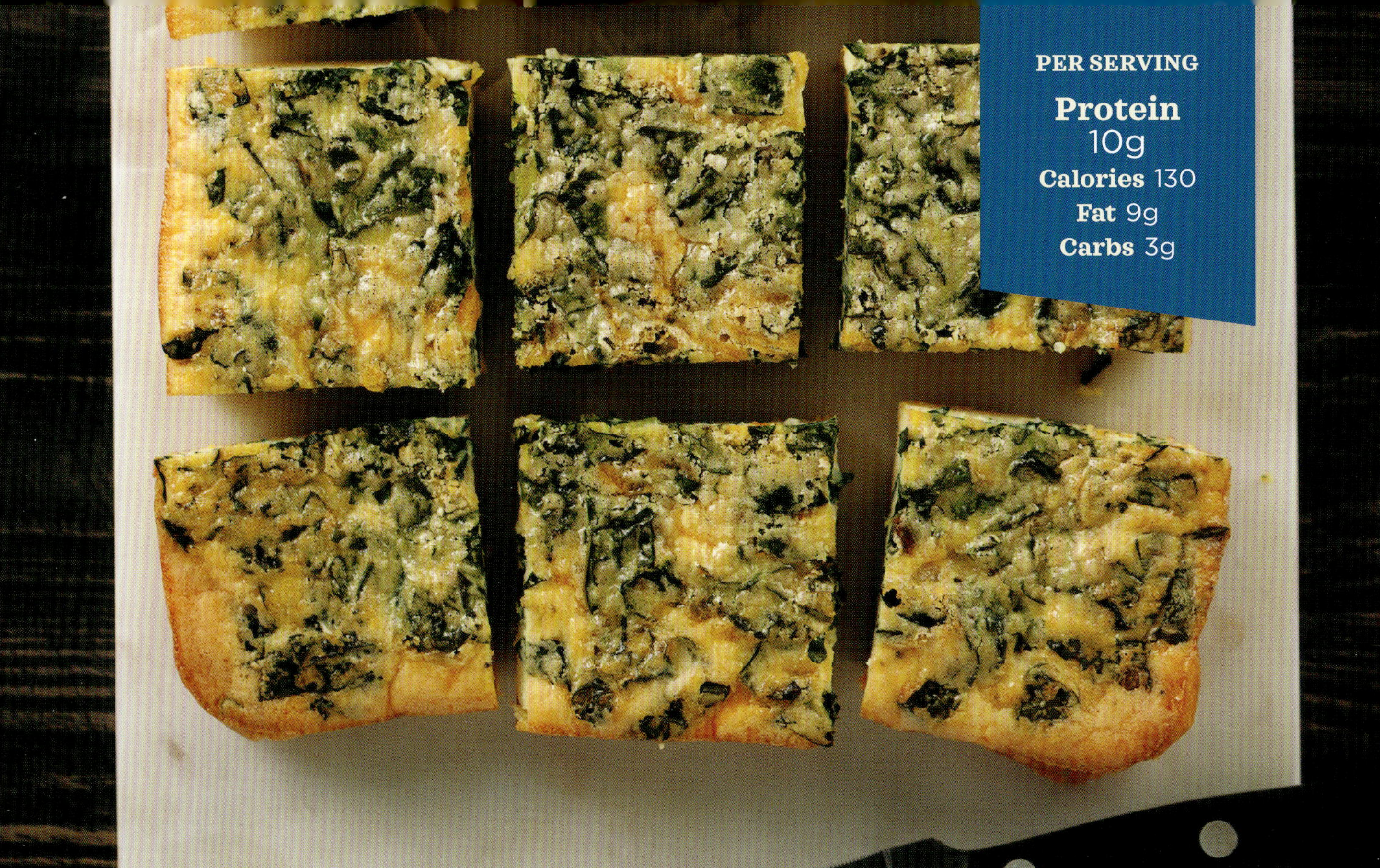

No-Crust Kale Quiche

MAKES 4 TO 6 SERVINGS

- 1 tablespoon olive oil
- 1 small onion, chopped
- 1 clove garlic, minced
- 3 to 4 ounces lacinato kale, cut into thin strips (about 1½ cups packed)
- ¾ teaspoon salt, divided
- 8 eggs
- 1 cup (4 ounces) grated Cheddar cheese
- ¾ cup whipping cream
- ¼ teaspoon black pepper

1. Preheat oven to 350°F. Spray 8-inch square baking pan with nonstick cooking spray.
2. Heat oil in medium skillet over medium-high heat. Add onion; cook and stir 3 minutes or until softened. Add garlic; cook and stir 1 minute. Add kale and ¼ teaspoon salt; cook over medium heat 10 minutes, stirring occasionally. Set aside to cool slightly.
3. Whisk eggs, cheese, cream, remaining ½ teaspoon salt and pepper in medium bowl until well blended. Stir in kale mixture. Pour into prepared pan.
4. Bake 30 to 35 minutes or until toothpick inserted into center comes out clean. Remove to wire rack; let stand 10 minutes before serving.

Zucchini-Tomato Frittata

MAKES 4 SERVINGS

- 1 cup sliced zucchini
- 1 cup broccoli florets
- 1 cup diced red or yellow bell pepper
- 3 whole eggs*
- 5 egg whites*
- ½ cup 1% low-fat cottage cheese
- ½ cup rehydrated** sun-dried tomatoes (1 ounce dry), coarsely chopped
- ¼ cup chopped green onions
- ¼ cup chopped fresh basil
- ⅛ teaspoon ground red pepper
- 2 tablespoons grated Parmesan cheese

**Or substitute 6 whole eggs or 1½ cups liquid egg substitute.*

***To rehydrate sun-dried tomatoes, pour 1 cup boiling water over tomatoes in small bowl. Let stand 5 to 10 minutes or until softened; drain well.*

1. Preheat broiler. Spray large ovenproof skillet with nonstick cooking spray; heat over medium-high heat. Add zucchini, broccoli and bell pepper; cook and stir 3 to 4 minutes or until vegetables are crisp-tender.

2. Whisk whole eggs, egg whites, cottage cheese, sun-dried tomatoes, green onions, basil and ground red pepper in medium bowl until well blended.

3. Pour over vegetables in skillet. Cook over medium heat 7 to 8 minutes or until frittata is almost firm and golden brown on bottom, gently lifting sides of frittata so uncooked egg flows underneath. Remove from heat; sprinkle with cheese.

4. Broil about 5 inches from heat source 3 to 5 minutes or until top begins to brown.

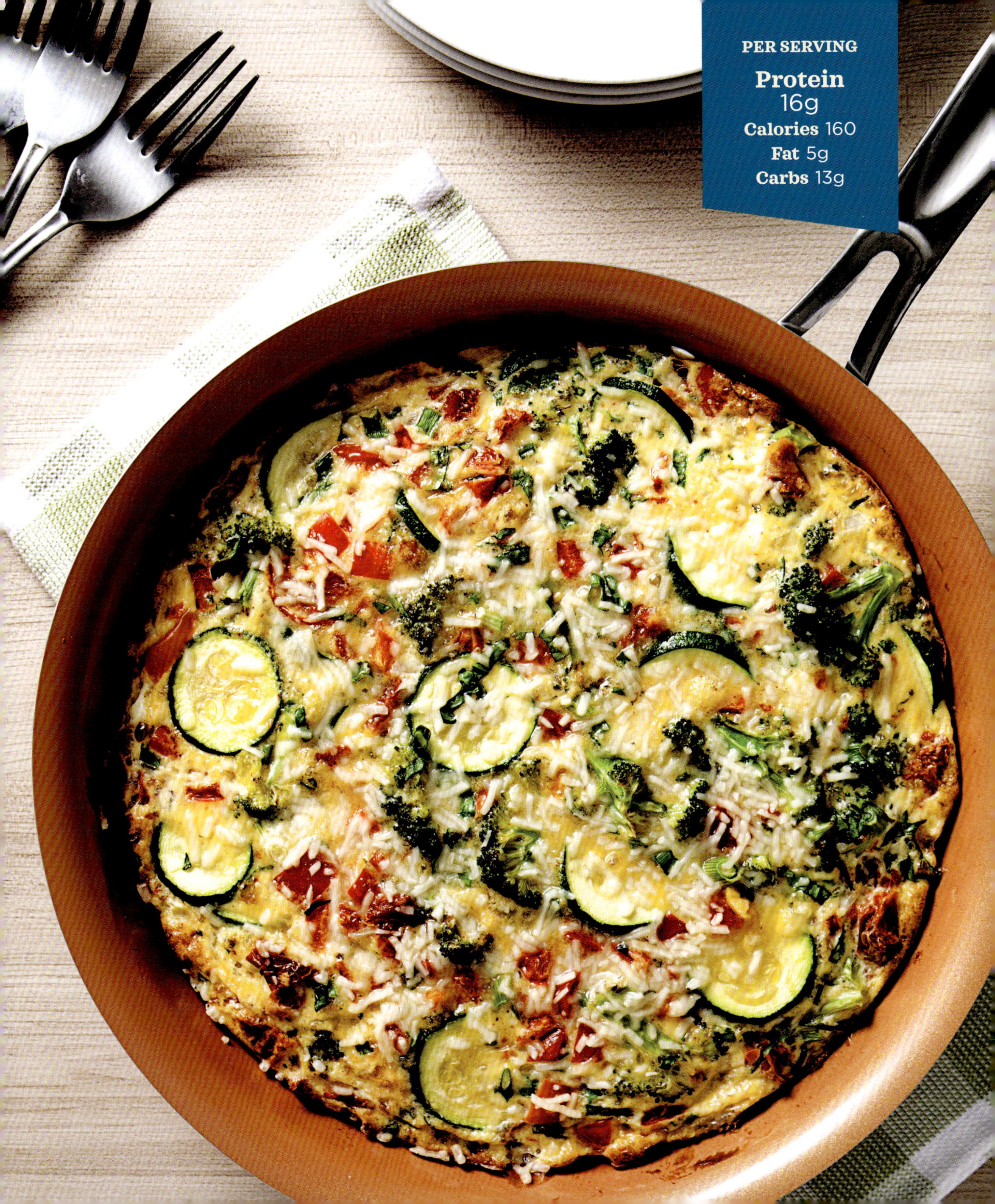
PER SERVING
Protein
16g
Calories 160
Fat 5g
Carbs 13g

Roasted Pepper and Sourdough Brunch Casserole

MAKES 8 SERVINGS

- **3 cups sourdough bread cubes**
- **1 jar (12 ounces) roasted red pepper strips, drained**
- **1 cup (4 ounces) shredded reduced-fat sharp Cheddar cheese**
- **1 cup (4 ounces) shredded reduced-fat Monterey Jack cheese**
- **1 cup fat-free cottage cheese**
- **1½ cups liquid egg substitute**
- **1 cup fat-free (skim) milk**
- **¼ cup chopped fresh cilantro**
- **¼ teaspoon black pepper**

1. Spray 11×7-inch baking dish with nonstick cooking spray. Spread bread cubes in prepared baking dish; top with roasted peppers, Cheddar and Monterey Jack.

2. Process cottage cheese in food processor or blender until smooth. Add egg substitute and milk; process just until blended. Pour over ingredients in baking dish; sprinkle with cilantro and black pepper. Cover and refrigerate 4 hours or overnight.

3. Preheat oven to 375°F. Bake, uncovered, 40 minutes or until center is set and top is lightly browned.

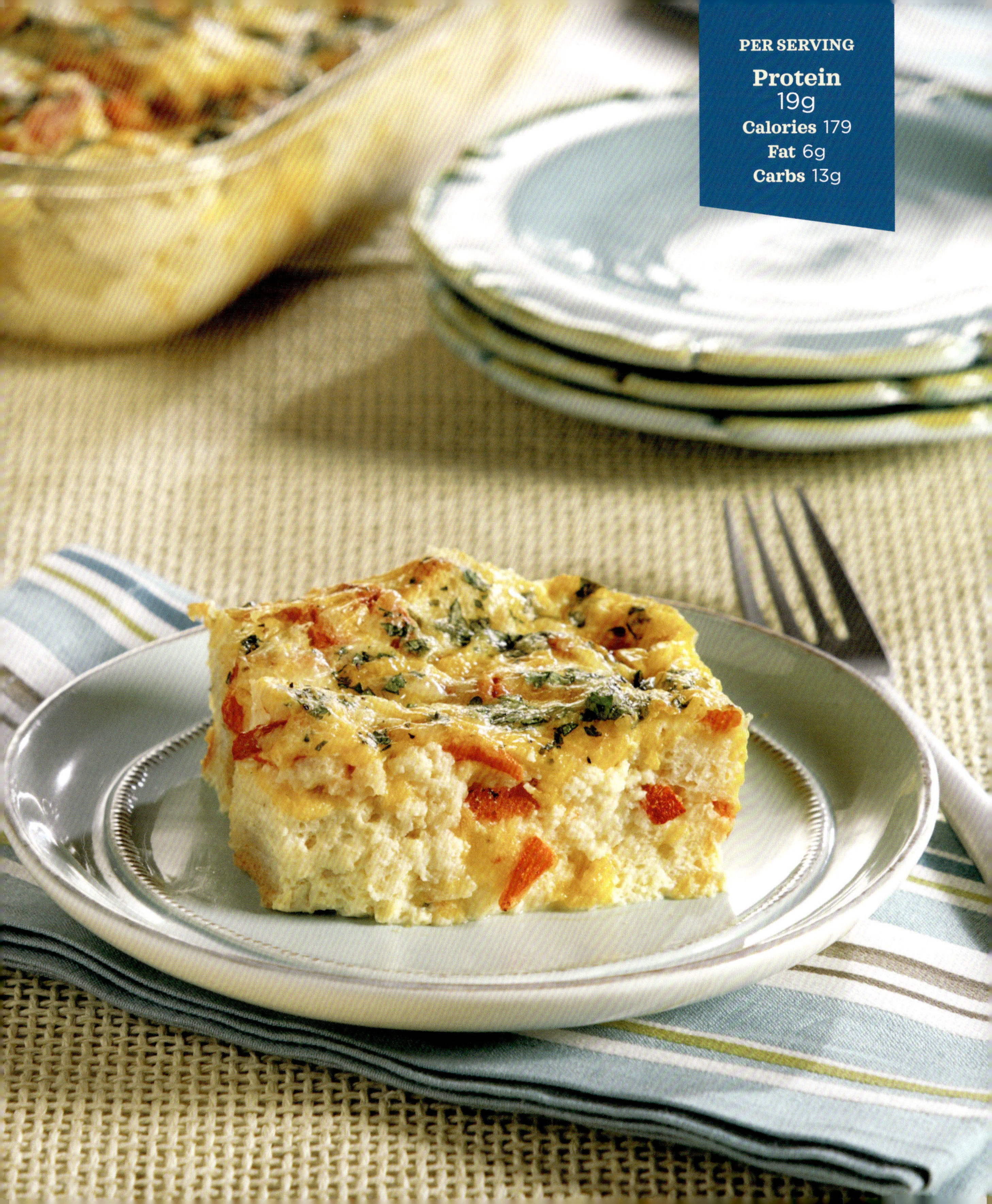

PER SERVING

Protein 19g

Calories 179

Fat 6g

Carbs 13g

Mini Spinach Frittatas

MAKES 4 SERVINGS (12 MINI FRITTATAS)

- 1 tablespoon olive oil
- ½ cup chopped onion
- 8 eggs
- ¼ cup plain yogurt
- 1 package (10 ounces) frozen chopped spinach, thawed and squeezed dry
- ½ cup (2 ounces) shredded white Cheddar cheese
- ¼ cup grated Parmesan cheese
- ¾ teaspoon salt
- ⅛ teaspoon black pepper
- ⅛ teaspoon ground red pepper
- Pinch ground nutmeg

1. Preheat oven to 350°F. Spray 12 standard (2½-inch) muffin cups with nonstick cooking spray.

2. Heat oil in medium skillet over medium heat. Add onion; cook and stir about 5 minutes or until tender. Set aside to cool slightly.

3. Whisk eggs and yogurt in large bowl. Stir in spinach, Cheddar, Parmesan, salt, black pepper, red pepper, nutmeg and onion until blended. Divide mixture evenly among prepared muffin cups.

4. Bake 20 to 25 minutes or until eggs are puffed, firm and no longer shiny. Cool in pan 2 minutes. Loosen bottom and sides with small spatula or knife; remove to wire rack. Serve warm, cold or at room temperature.

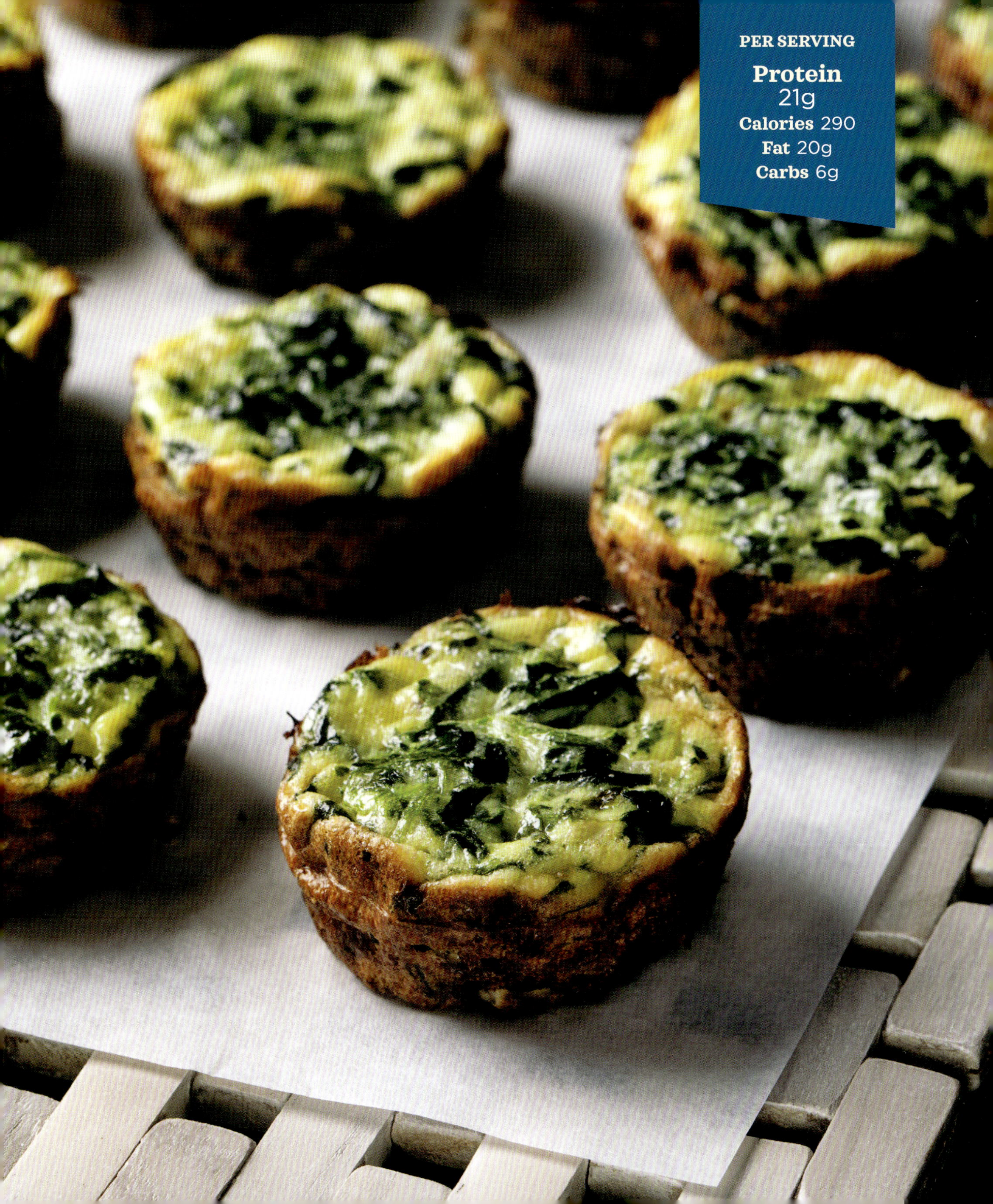
PER SERVING
Protein
21g
Calories 290
Fat 20g
Carbs 6g

PER SERVING
Protein
10g
Calories 340
Fat 16g
Carbs 45g

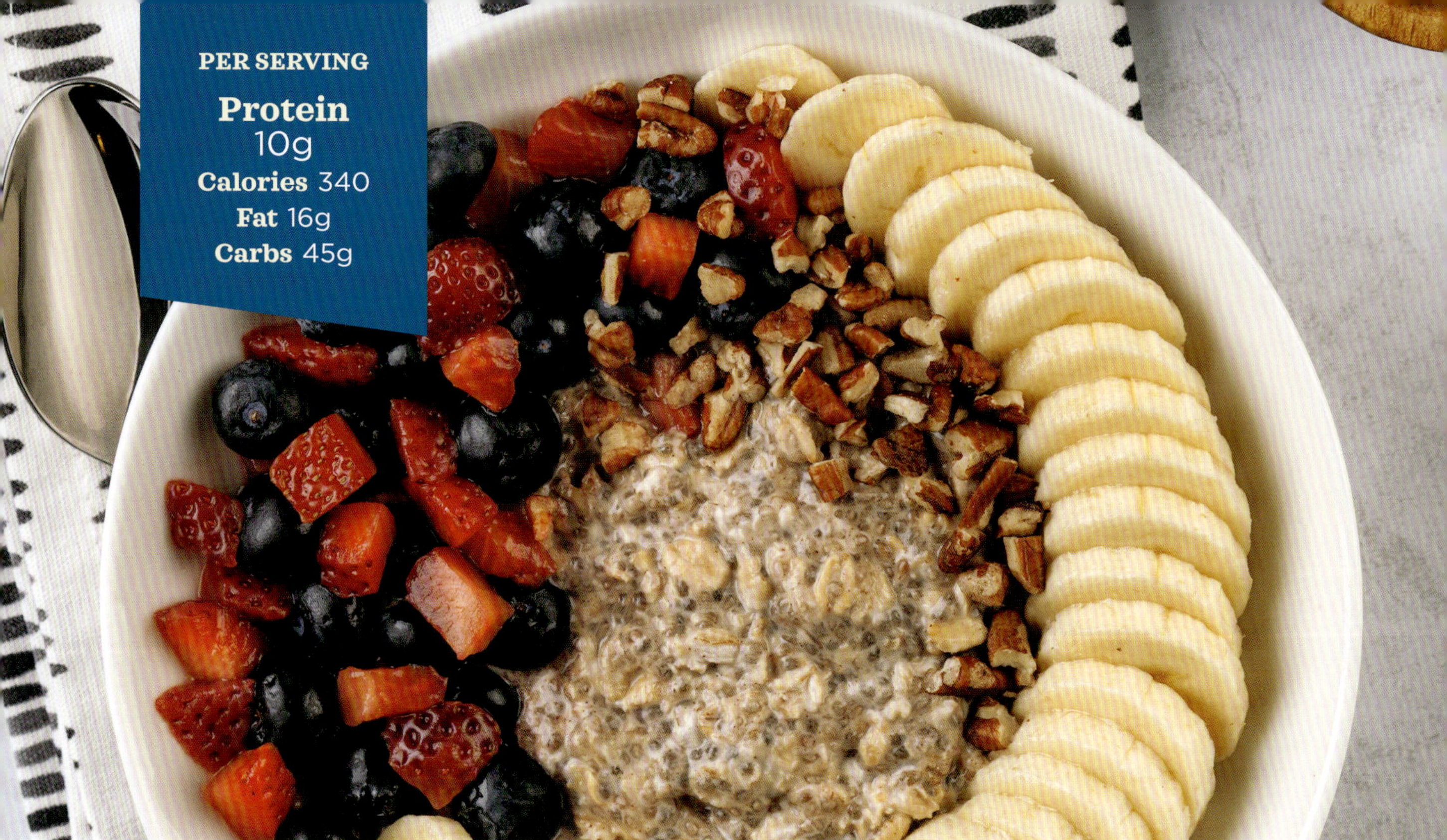

Overnight Chia Oat Pudding

MAKES 4 SERVINGS

- 1 cup old-fashioned oats
- ¼ cup chia seeds
- 3 tablespoons palm sugar or packed brown sugar, divided
- ½ teaspoon ground cinnamon
- ½ teaspoon salt
- 1¾ cups oatmilk
- 1 cup fresh strawberries, stemmed and diced
- 1 cup fresh blueberries
- 4 tablespoons chopped pecans or sliced almonds
- 4 bananas, sliced (optional)

1 Combine oats, chia seeds, 2 tablespoons sugar, cinnamon and salt in medium bowl or food storage container. Add oatmilk; stir until well blended. Cover and refrigerate overnight.

2 Combine strawberries and remaining 1 tablespoon sugar in another medium bowl or food storage container. Cover and refrigerate overnight.

3 Stir oat mixture. Stir blueberries into strawberries. For each serving, scoop ½ cup oat mixture into bowl. Top with strawberry mixture, blueberries and pecans. Serve with bananas, if desired.

PER SERVING
Protein
17g
Calories 187
Fat 11g
Carbs 4g
17g

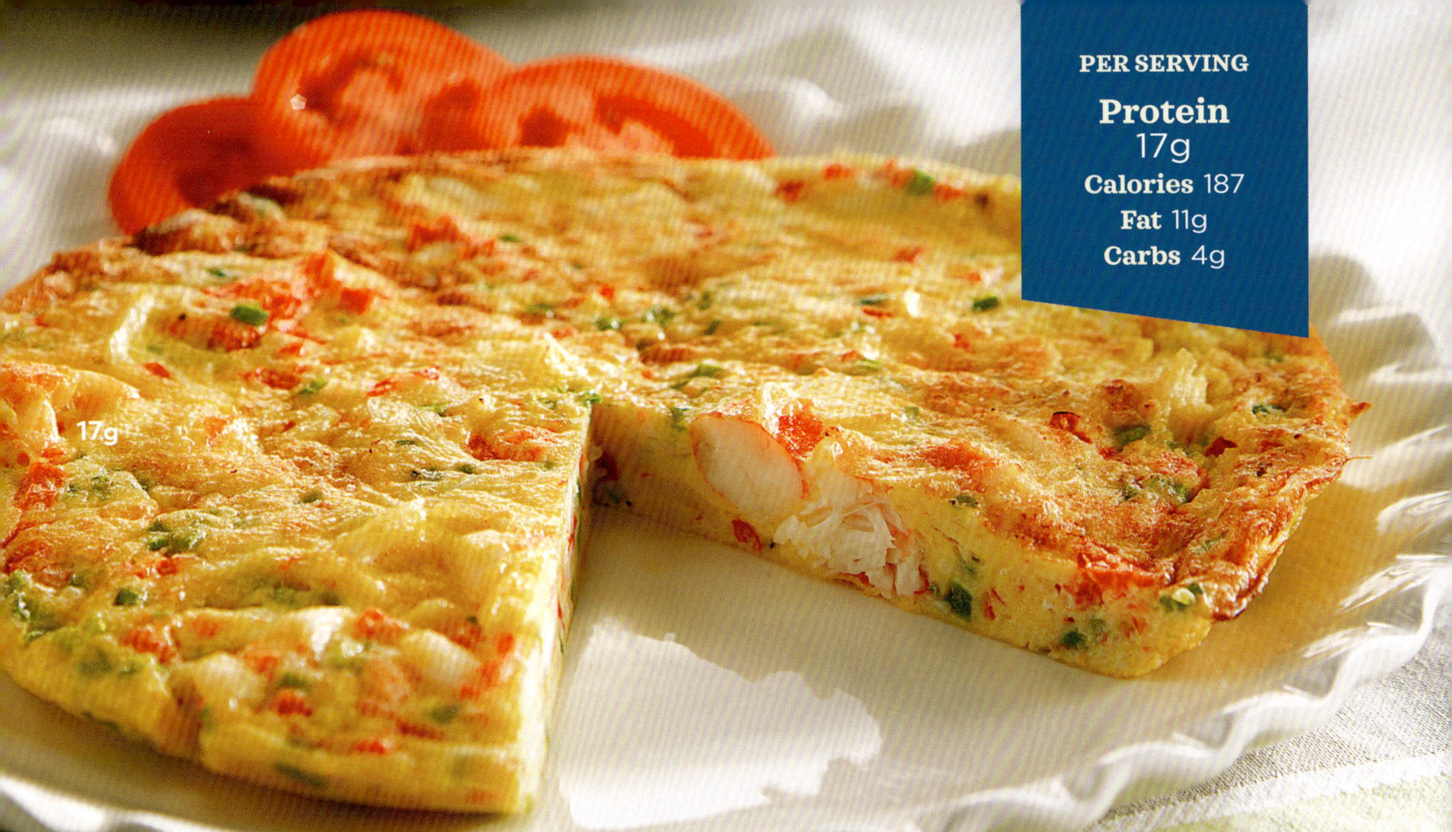

Spicy Crabmeat Frittata

MAKES 4 SERVINGS

- 1 can (about 6 ounces) lump white crabmeat, drained
- 6 eggs
- ¼ teaspoon salt
- ¼ teaspoon black pepper
- ¼ teaspoon hot pepper sauce
- 1 tablespoon olive oil
- 1 green bell pepper, finely chopped
- 2 cloves garlic, minced
- 1 plum tomato, seeded and finely chopped

1. Preheat broiler. Pick out and discard any shell or cartilage from crabmeat; break up large pieces of crabmeat.

2. Beat eggs in medium bowl. Add crabmeat, salt, black pepper and hot pepper sauce; stir until blended.

3. Heat oil in large broilerproof skillet over medium-high heat. Add bell pepper and garlic; cook and stir 3 minutes or until tender. Add tomato; cook and stir 1 minute. Stir in egg mixture; cook over medium-low heat 7 minutes or until eggs begin to set around edges.

4. Broil about 4 inches from heat source 1 to 2 minutes or until frittata is golden brown and center is set.

Smoked Salmon Omelet

MAKES 1 SERVING

- 3 eggs
- 2 tablespoons milk
- 1 tablespoon grated Parmesan cheese
- Pinch white or black pepper
- 1 teaspoon butter
- 2 tablespoons finely chopped red onion, divided
- 1 ounce smoked salmon, cut into 1- to 2-inch pieces
- 2 tablespoons sour cream
- 1 tablespoon water
- 1 tablespoon capers, rinsed and drained
- Finely chopped fresh parsley (optional)

1 Whisk eggs, milk, cheese and pepper in small bowl until well blended.

2 Melt butter in small (6-inch) nonstick skillet over medium-high heat. Pour egg mixture into skillet; stir briefly. Let eggs begin to set at edges, then lift edges and tilt skillet, allowing uncooked portion of egg mixture to flow underneath. Cook 1 minute or until omelet begins to set. Sprinkle 1 tablespoon onion over half of omelet; top with smoked salmon. Fold other half of omelet over filling; cook 1 minute. Slide omelet onto serving plate.

3 Whisk sour cream and water in small bowl until blended. Drizzle over omelet; top with remaining 1 tablespoon onion, capers and parsley, if desired.

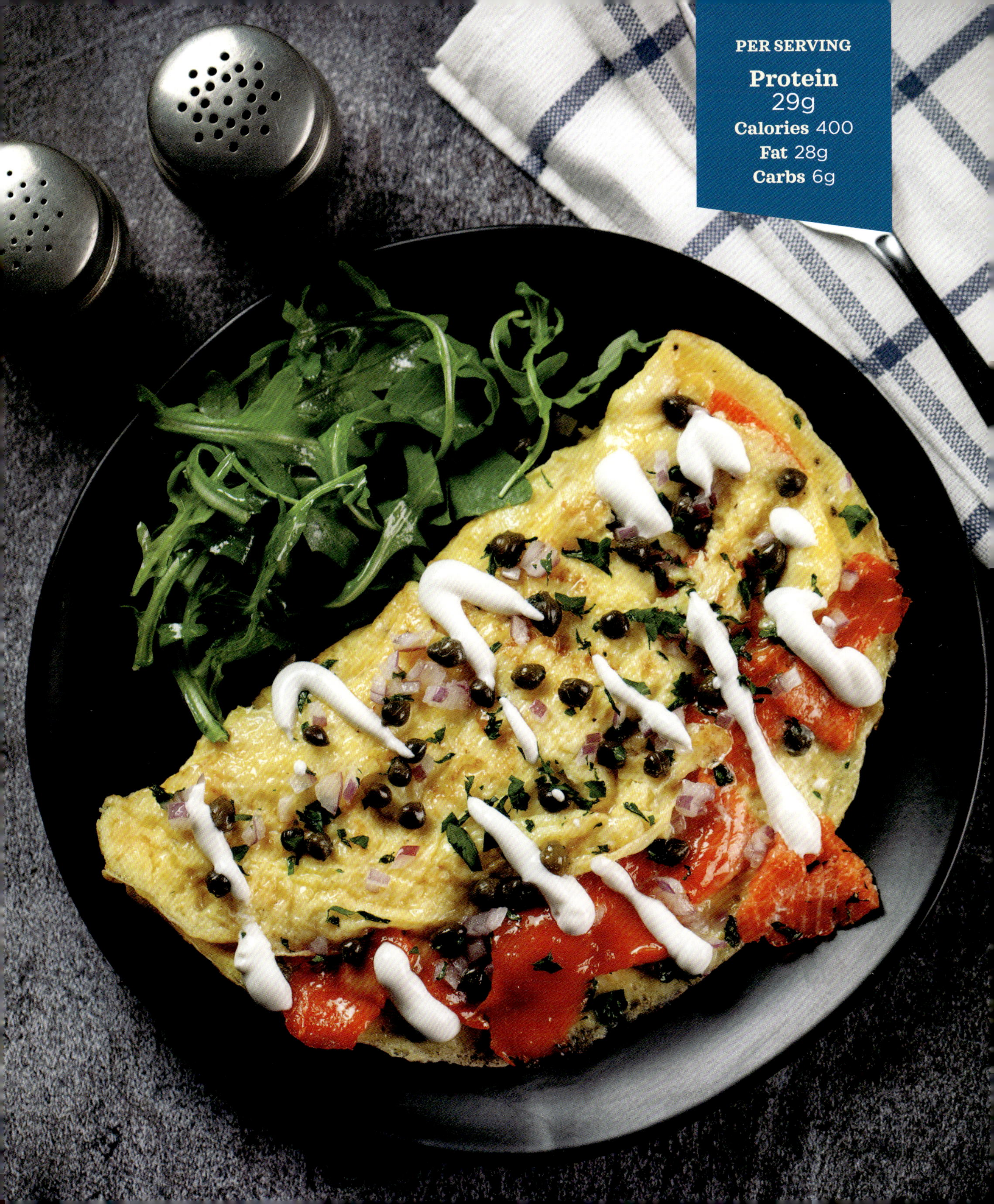
PER SERVING
Protein
29g
Calories 400
Fat 28g
Carbs 6g

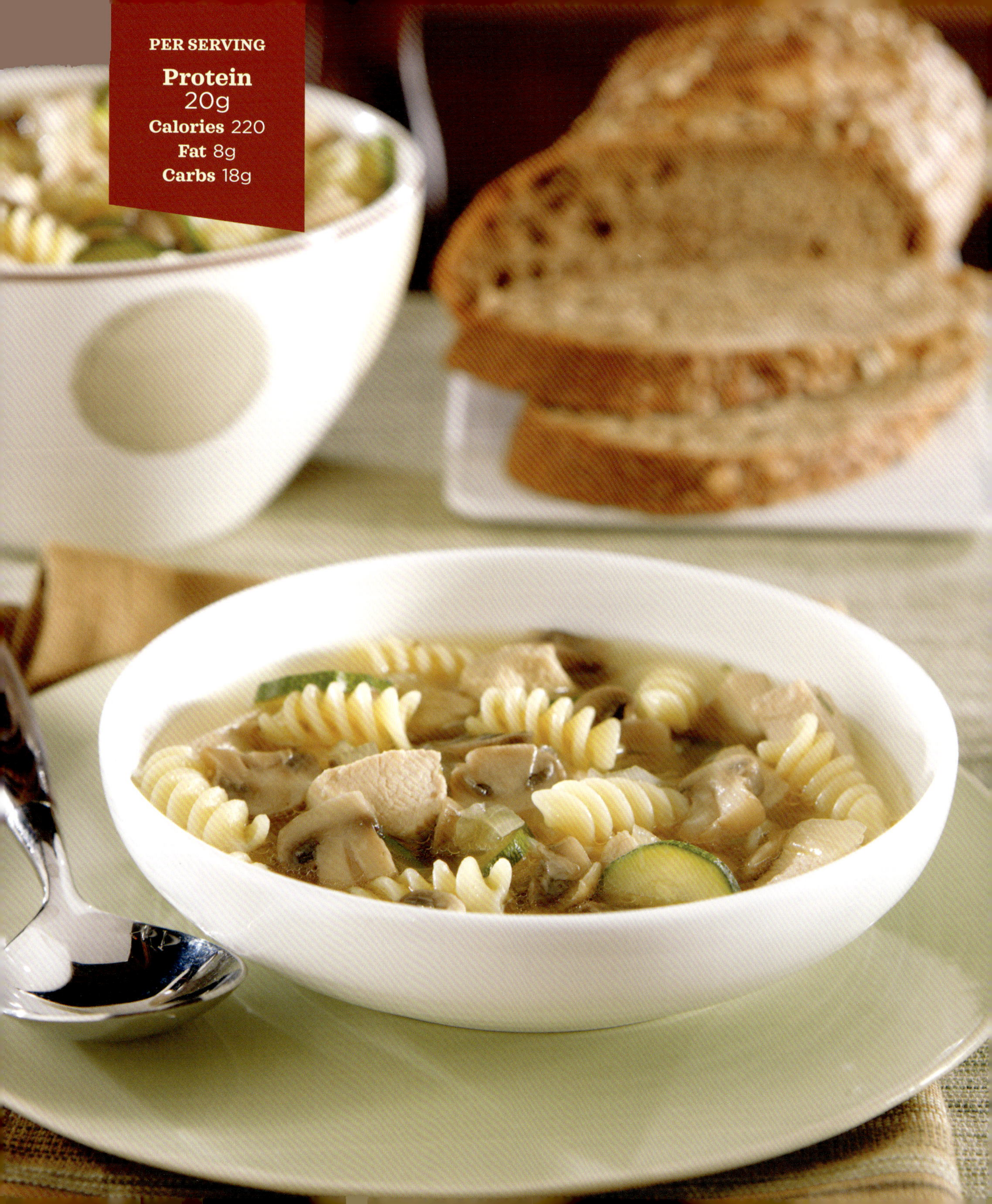
PER SERVING
Protein
20g
Calories 220
Fat 8g
Carbs 18g

SOUPS

Chicken Rotini Soup

MAKES 4 SERVINGS

- 2 tablespoons butter
- 8 ounces boneless skinless chicken breasts, cut into ½-inch pieces
- ½ medium onion, chopped
- 4 ounces mushrooms, sliced
- 4 cups reduced-sodium chicken broth
- 1 teaspoon Worcestershire sauce
- ¼ teaspoon dried tarragon
- ¾ cup uncooked rotini pasta
- 1 small zucchini, cut into thin (⅛-inch) slices

1 Melt butter in large saucepan or Dutch oven over medium heat. Add chicken, onion and mushrooms; cook and stir 5 minutes or until onion is softened and chicken is lightly browned.

2 Stir in broth, Worcestershire sauce and tarragon; bring to a boil over high heat. Stir in pasta. Reduce heat to medium-low; simmer, uncovered, 5 minutes, stirring occasionally.

3 Add zucchini to soup; cook about 5 minutes or until pasta is tender.

Chickpea Vegetable Soup

MAKES 4 SERVINGS

- 1 teaspoon olive oil
- 1 cup chopped onion
- ½ cup chopped green bell pepper
- 2 cloves garlic, minced
- 2 cans (about 14 ounces each) diced tomatoes
- 3 cups water
- 2 cups broccoli florets
- 1 can (about 15 ounces) chickpeas, rinsed, drained and slightly mashed
- ½ cup (3 ounces) uncooked orzo or rosamarina pasta
- 1 bay leaf
- 1 tablespoon chopped fresh thyme *or* 1 teaspoon dried thyme
- 1 tablespoon chopped fresh rosemary *or* 1 teaspoon dried rosemary
- 1 tablespoon lime or lemon juice
- ½ teaspoon ground turmeric
- ¼ teaspoon salt
- ¼ teaspoon ground red pepper
- ¼ cup pumpkin seeds or sunflower kernels

1. Heat oil in large saucepan over medium heat. Add onion, bell pepper and garlic; cook and stir 5 minutes or until vegetables are tender.

2. Add tomatoes, water, broccoli, chickpeas, orzo, bay leaf, thyme, rosemary, lime juice, turmeric, salt and ground red pepper; bring to a boil over high heat. Reduce heat to medium-low; cover and simmer 10 to 12 minutes or until orzo is tender.

3. Remove and discard bay leaf. Sprinkle with pumpkin seeds.

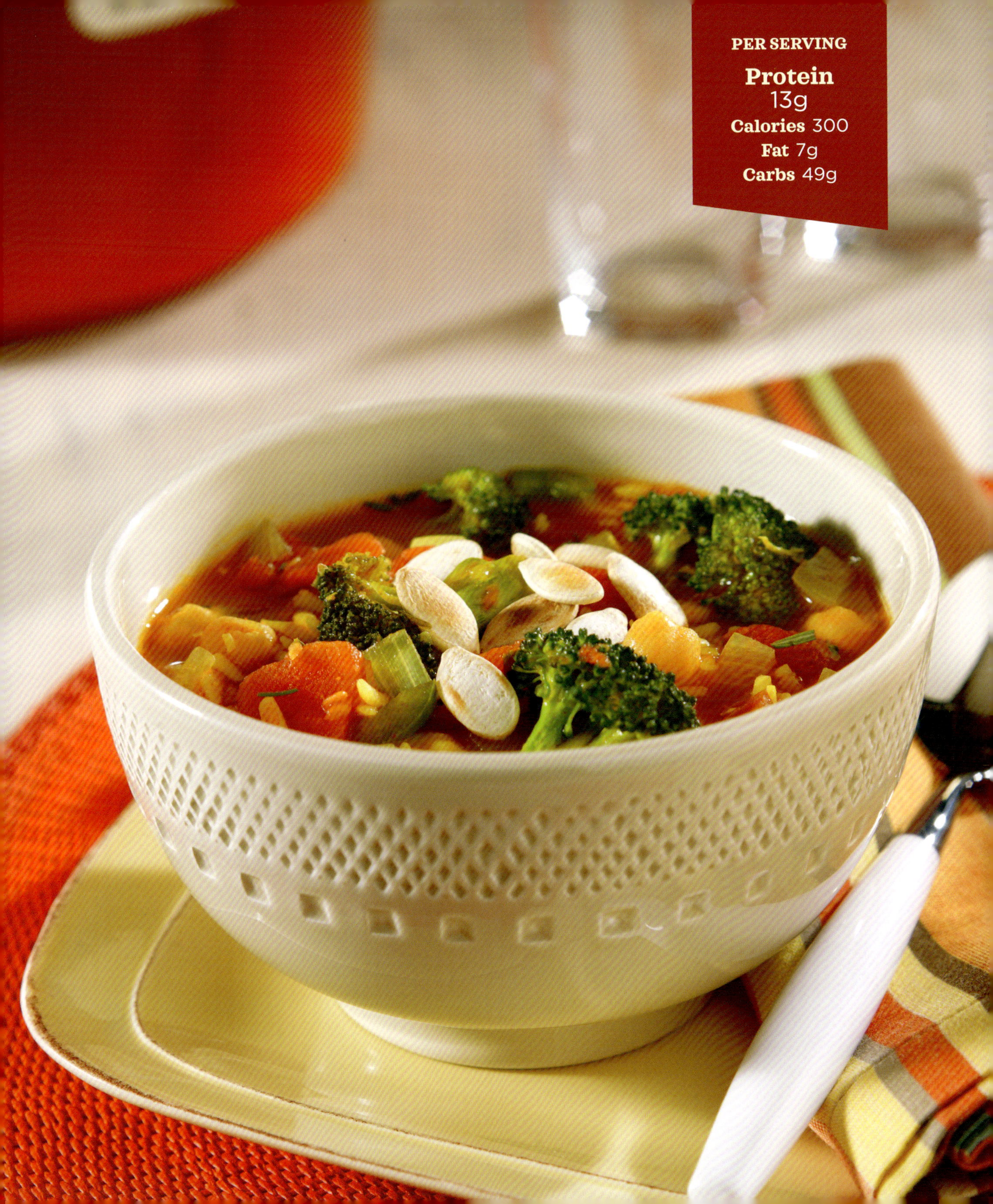
PER SERVING
Protein
13g
Calories 300
Fat 7g
Carbs 49g

Cioppino

MAKES 4 SERVINGS

- 1 teaspoon olive oil
- 1 large onion, chopped
- 1 cup sliced celery
- 1 clove garlic, minced
- 4 cups water
- 1 tablespoon Italian seasoning
- 1 cube fish-flavored bouillon
- 4 ounces cod or other boneless mild-flavored fish fillets, cut into ½-inch pieces
- 1 large tomato, chopped
- 1 can (10 ounces) baby clams, rinsed and drained (optional)
- 4 ounces small raw shrimp, peeled and deveined
- 4 ounces raw bay scallops
- ¼ cup flaked crabmeat or crabmeat blend
- 2 tablespoons lemon juice

1. Heat oil in large saucepan over medium heat. Add onion, celery and garlic; cook and stir 5 minutes or until onion is soft.

2. Add water, Italian seasoning and bouillon; bring to a boil over high heat. Stir in fish and tomato. Reduce heat to medium-low; simmer about 5 minutes or until fish is opaque.

3. Add clams, if desired, shrimp, scallops, crabmeat and lemon juice; simmer about 5 minutes or until shrimp and scallops are opaque.

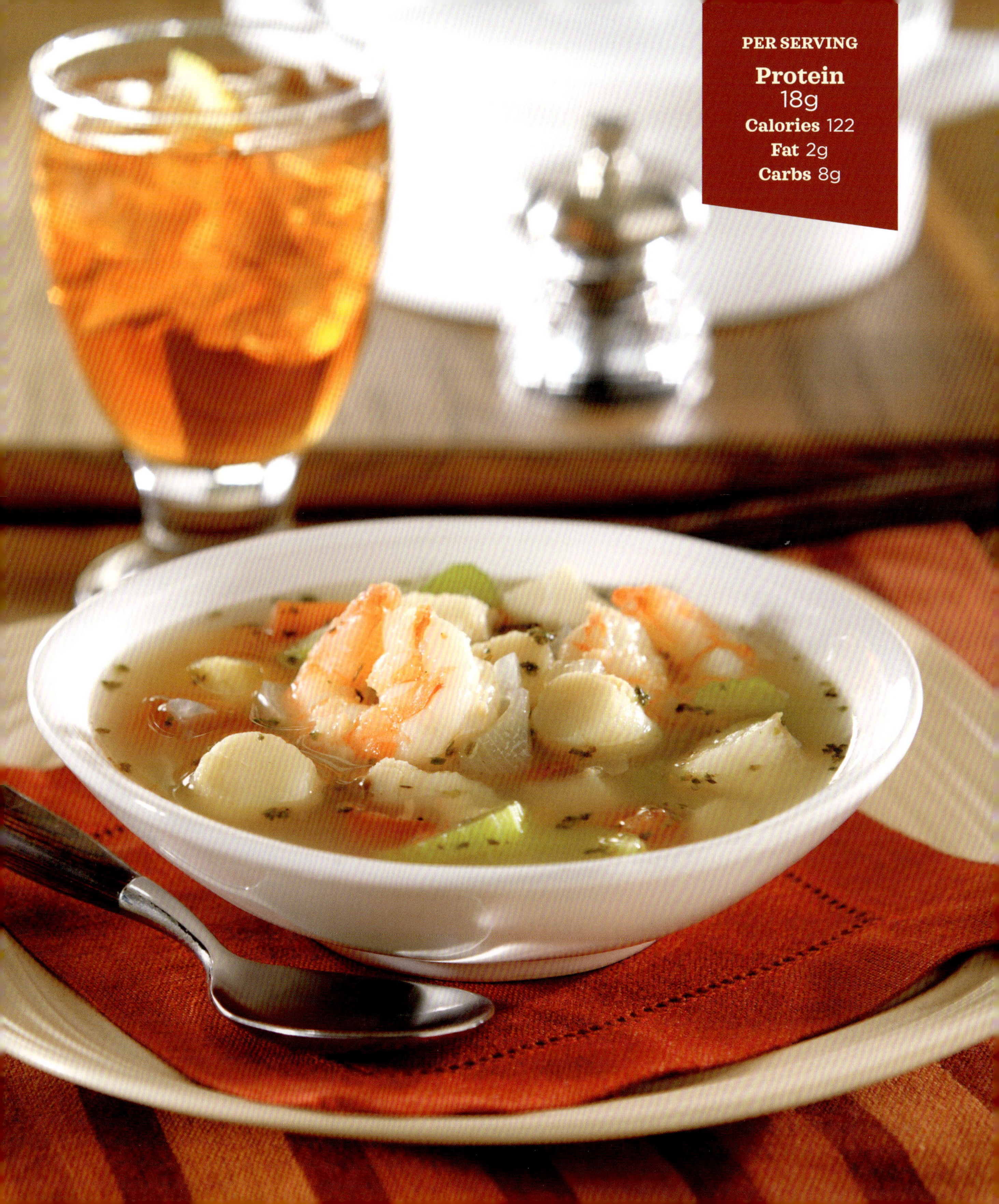

PER SERVING
Protein
18g
Calories 122
Fat 2g
Carbs 8g

Middle Eastern Lentil Soup

MAKES 4 SERVINGS

- 2 tablespoons olive oil
- 1 small onion, chopped
- 1 medium red bell pepper, chopped
- 1 teaspoon whole fennel seeds
- ½ teaspoon ground cumin
- ¼ teaspoon ground red pepper
- 4 cups water
- 1 cup dried lentils, rinsed and sorted
- ½ teaspoon salt
- 1 tablespoon lemon juice
- ½ cup plain low-fat yogurt
- 2 tablespoons chopped fresh parsley

1. Heat oil in large saucepan over medium-high heat. Add onion and bell pepper; cook and stir 5 minutes or until vegetables are tender. Add fennel seeds, cumin and ground red pepper; cook and stir 1 minute.

2. Stir in water, lentils and salt; bring to a boil. Reduce heat to low; cover and simmer 25 to 30 minutes or until lentils are tender. Stir in lemon juice.

3. Top each serving with yogurt; sprinkle with parsley.

Tip

Serve with homemade pita chips. Cut four pita bread rounds into six wedges each. Toss wedges with 1 tablespoon olive oil and 1 teaspoon coarse salt; spread on baking sheet. Bake at 350°F 15 minutes or until lightly browned and crisp.

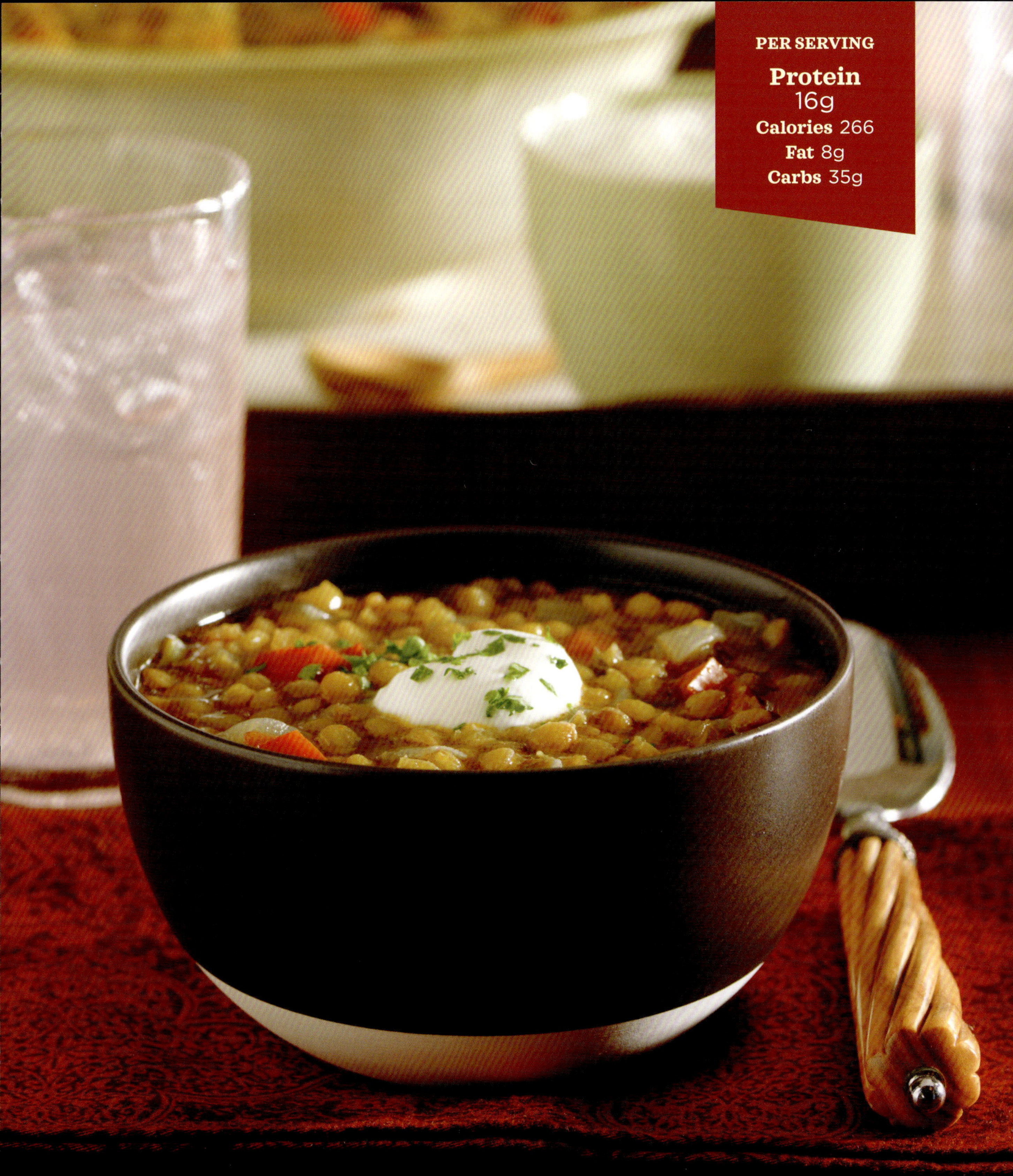
PER SERVING
Protein
16g
Calories 266
Fat 8g
Carbs 35g

Southwest Corn and Turkey Soup

MAKES 6 SERVINGS

- 2 dried ancho chiles (each about 4 inches long) *or* 6 dried New Mexico chiles (about 6 inches long)
- 1 medium onion, thinly sliced
- 3 cloves garlic, minced
- 1 teaspoon ground cumin
- 3 cans (about 14 ounces each) reduced-sodium chicken broth
- 2 small zucchini, cut into ½-inch slices
- 1½ to 2 cups shredded cooked turkey or chicken
- 1 can (about 15 ounces) black beans or chickpeas, rinsed and drained
- 1 package (10 ounces) frozen corn
- ¼ cup yellow cornmeal
- 1 teaspoon dried oregano
- ⅓ cup chopped fresh cilantro

1. Cut stems from chiles; remove and discard seeds. Place chiles in medium bowl; cover with boiling water. Let stand 20 to 40 minutes or until chiles are softened.

2. Drain chiles; cut open lengthwise and lay flat on work surface. Scrape chile pulp from skins with edge of small knife. Finely mince pulp; discard skins.

3. Spray large saucepan with nonstick cooking spray; heat over medium heat. Add onion; cook and stir 4 minutes. Add garlic and cumin; cook and stir 30 seconds.

4. Stir in broth, chile pulp, zucchini, turkey, beans, corn, cornmeal and oregano; bring to a boil over high heat. Reduce heat to low; simmer 15 minutes or until zucchini is tender. Stir in cilantro just before serving.

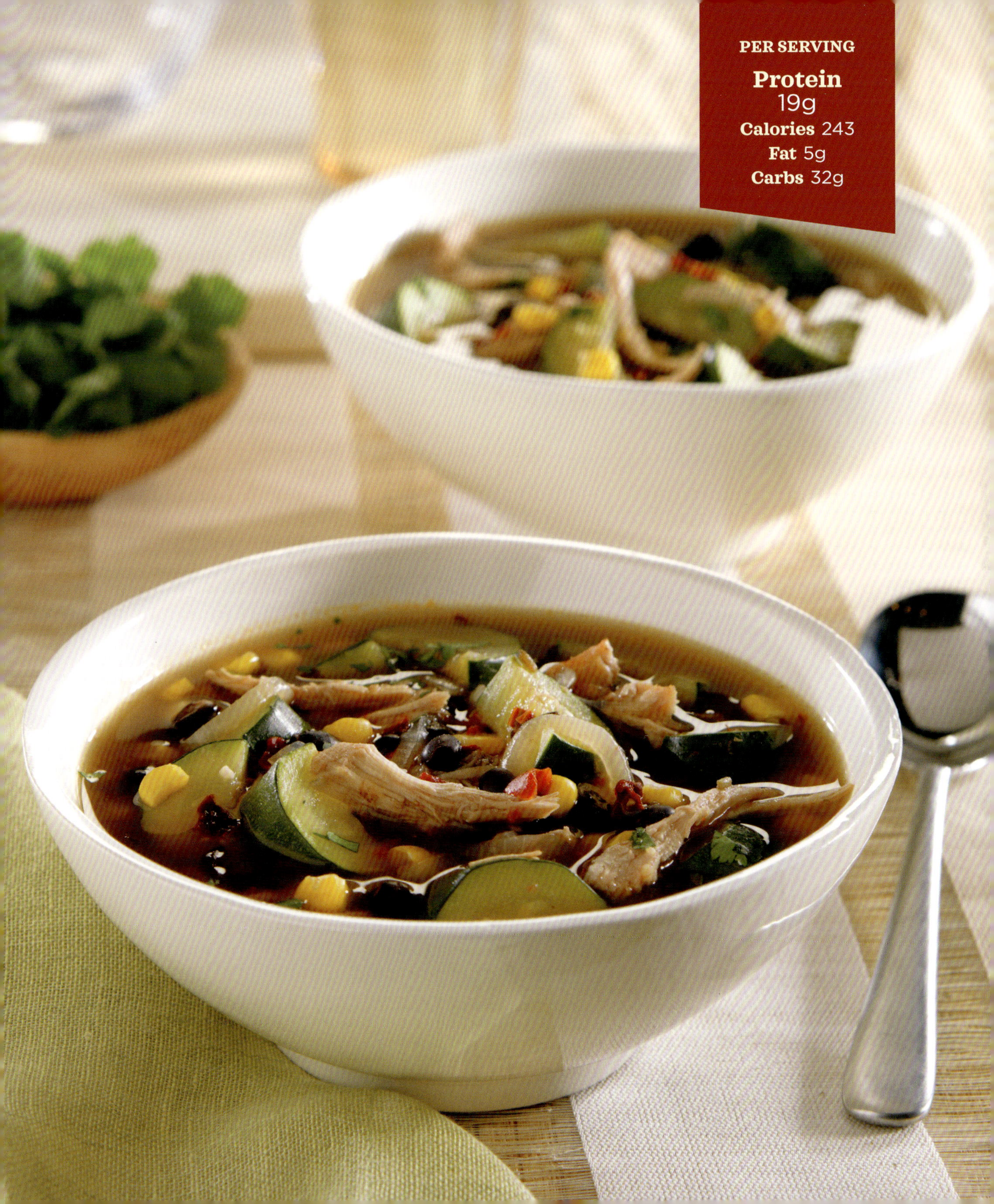
PER SERVING
Protein
19g
Calories 243
Fat 5g
Carbs 32g

Ground Beef, Spinach and Barley Soup

MAKES 4 SERVINGS

- 12 ounces 95% lean ground beef
- 4 cups water
- 1 can (about 14 ounces) stewed tomatoes
- 1½ cups thinly sliced carrots
- 1 cup chopped onion
- ½ cup quick-cooking pearl barley
- 1½ teaspoons beef bouillon granules
- 1½ teaspoons dried thyme
- 1 teaspoon dried oregano
- ½ teaspoon garlic powder
- ¼ teaspoon black pepper
- ⅛ teaspoon salt
- 3 cups fresh spinach leaves

1. Cook beef in large saucepan over medium-high heat 6 to 8 minutes or until browned, stirring to break up meat. Rinse beef under warm water; drain.

2. Return beef to saucepan; stir in 4 cups water, tomatoes, carrots, onion, barley, bouillon, thyme, oregano, garlic powder, pepper and salt; bring to a boil over high heat. Reduce heat to medium-low; cover and simmer 12 to 15 minutes or until barley and vegetables are tender, stirring occasionally.

3. Stir in spinach; cook just until spinach begins to wilt.

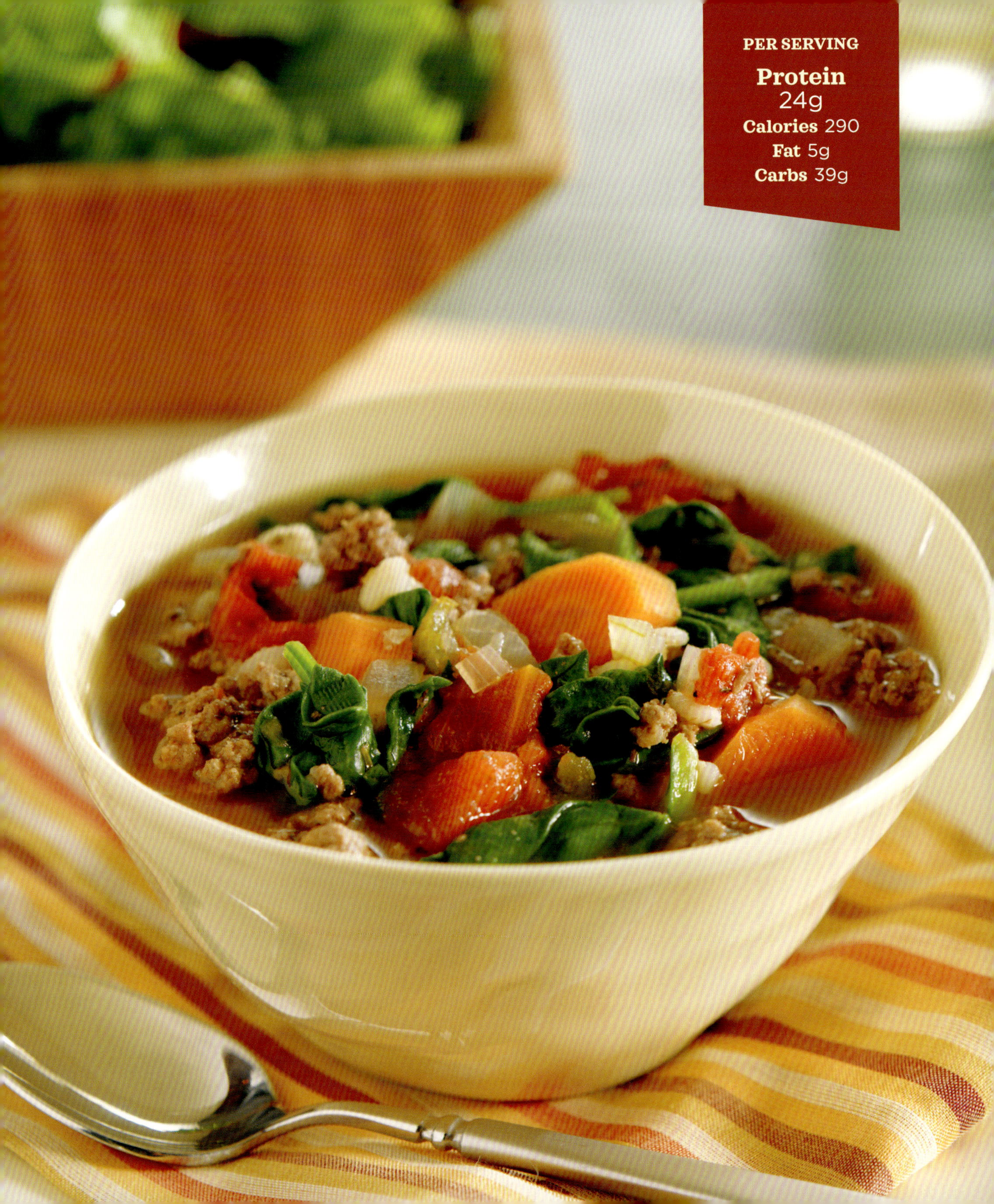
PER SERVING
Protein
24g
Calories 290
Fat 5g
Carbs 39g

Italian-Style Bean Soup

MAKES 8 TO 10 SERVINGS

- **1½ cups dried Great Northern or navy beans, rinsed and sorted**
- **5 to 6 cups water**
- **1 cup pasta sauce**
- **1 tablespoon dried minced onion**
- **2 teaspoons dried basil**
- **2 cubes chicken bouillon**
- **1 teaspoon dried parsley flakes**
- **½ teaspoon minced garlic**
- **1½ cups uncooked medium pasta shells**
- **8 ounces baby spinach (optional)**
- **Salt and black pepper**
- **¼ cup grated Parmesan cheese**

1 Place beans in large bowl; add water to cover. Soak 6 to 8 hours or overnight.*

2 Drain beans; discard water. Combine beans, 5 cups water, pasta sauce, onion, basil, bouillon, parsley flakes and garlic in large saucepan or Dutch oven; bring to a boil over high heat. Reduce heat to low; cover and simmer 2 to 2½ hours.

3 Add pasta and spinach, if desired; cover and simmer 15 to 20 minutes or until pasta is tender. Season with salt and pepper; sprinkle with cheese.

**To quick soak beans, place in large saucepan; add water to cover. Bring to a boil over high heat; boil 2 minutes. Remove from heat; let soak, covered, 1 hour.*

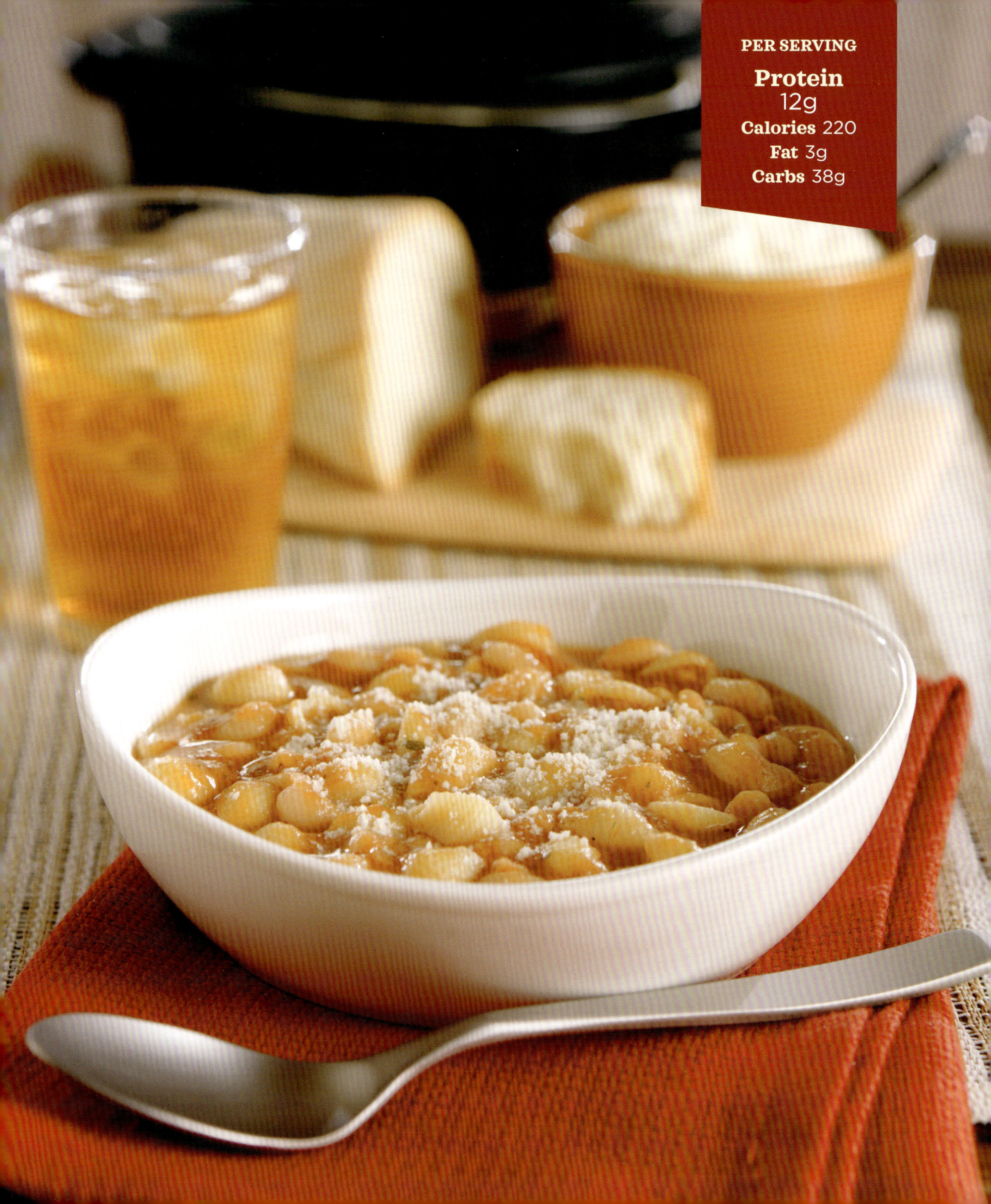
PER SERVING
Protein
12g
Calories 220
Fat 3g
Carbs 38g

North African Chicken Soup

MAKES 4 SERVINGS

- ¾ teaspoon paprika
- ½ teaspoon ground ginger
- ½ teaspoon ground cumin
- ½ teaspoon ground allspice
- 8 ounces boneless skinless chicken breasts, cut into bite-size pieces
- 2½ cups reduced-sodium chicken broth
- 2 cups peeled sweet potato, cut into ½-inch pieces
- 1 cup chopped onion
- ½ cup water
- 3 cloves garlic, minced
- 1 teaspoon sugar
- 2 cups undrained canned tomatoes, cut up
- Black pepper

1 Combine paprika, ginger, cumin and allspice in small bowl; mix well. Combine 1 teaspoon spice mixture and chicken in medium bowl; toss to coat.

2 Spray large saucepan with nonstick cooking spray; heat over medium-high heat. Add chicken; cook and stir 3 to 4 minutes or until cooked through. Remove to plate.

3 Add broth, sweet potato, onion, water, garlic, sugar and remaining spice mixture to saucepan; bring to a boil over high heat. Reduce heat to medium-low; cover and simmer 10 minutes or until sweet potato is tender.

4 Stir in tomatoes and chicken; cook until heated through. Season with pepper.

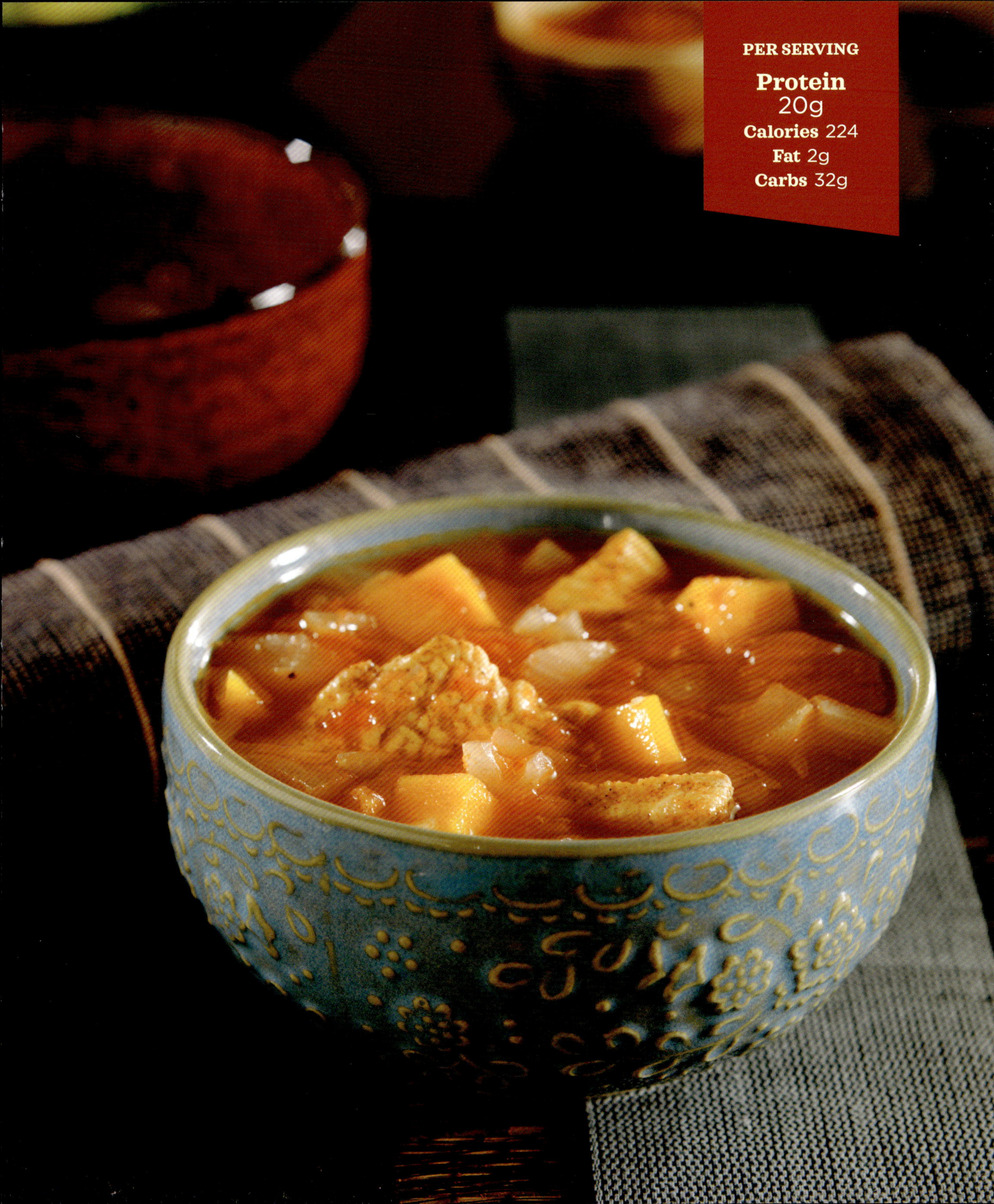
PER SERVING
Protein
20g
Calories 224
Fat 2g
Carbs 32g

Spicy Thai Shrimp Soup

MAKES 4 SERVINGS

- 1 tablespoon vegetable oil
- 1 pound medium raw shrimp, peeled and deveined, shells reserved
- 1 jalapeño pepper, cut into slivers
- 1 tablespoon paprika
- ¼ teaspoon ground red pepper
- 4 cans (about 14 ounces each) chicken broth
- 1 (½-inch) strip *each* lemon and lime peel
- 1 can (15 ounces) straw mushrooms, drained
- Juice of 1 lemon
- Juice of 1 lime
- 2 tablespoons soy sauce
- 1 red Thai pepper or red jalapeño pepper *or* ¼ small red bell pepper, cut into strips
- ¼ cup fresh cilantro leaves

1 Heat oil in large skillet or wok over medium-high heat. Add shrimp and jalapeño; cook and stir 1 minute. Add paprika and ground red pepper; cook and stir 1 minute or until shrimp are pink and opaque. Remove to medium bowl.

2 Add shrimp shells to skillet; cook and stir 30 seconds. Add broth and lemon and lime peels; bring to a boil. Reduce heat to low; cover and simmer 15 minutes.

3 Remove and discard shrimp shells and citrus peels with slotted spoon. Add mushrooms and shrimp to broth; bring to a boil over medium heat. Stir in lemon and lime juices, soy sauce and Thai pepper; cook and stir until heated through. Sprinkle with cilantro. Serve immediately.

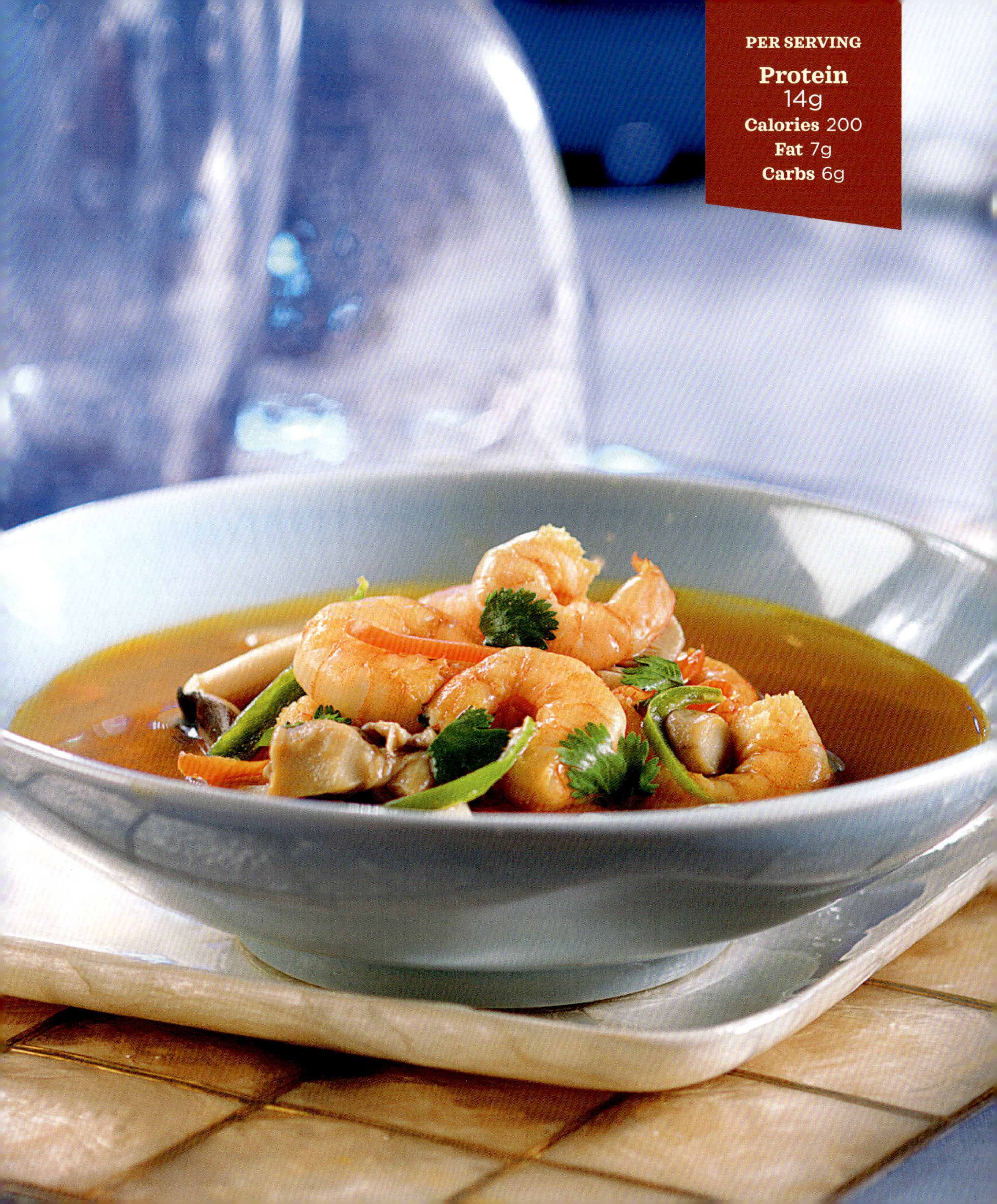

PER SERVING

Protein 14g
Calories 200
Fat 7g
Carbs 6g

PER SERVING

Protein
30g

Calories 450

Fat 12g

Carbs 54g

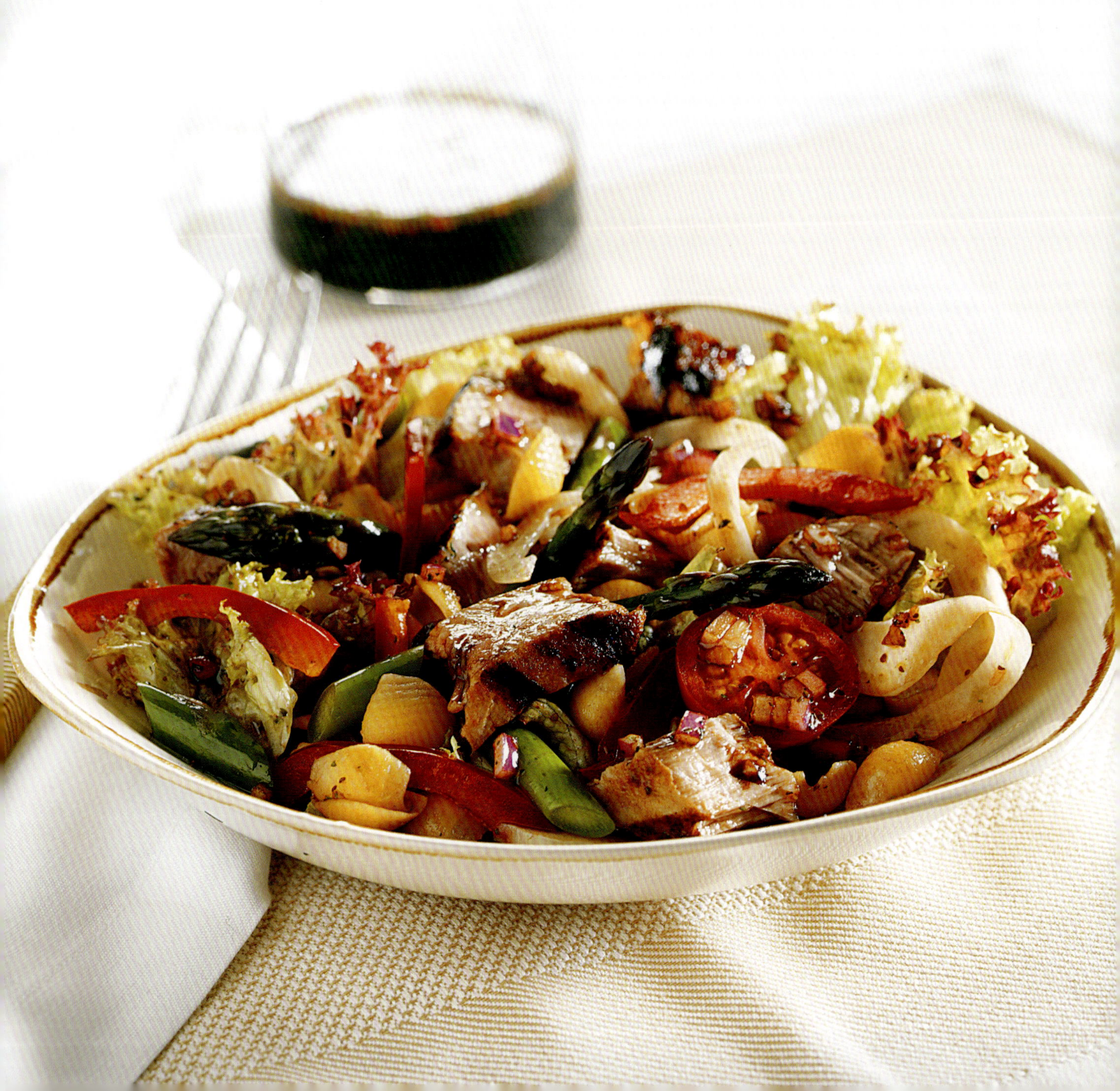

SALADS

Tuna, Fennel and Pasta Salad

MAKES 4 SERVINGS

- Balsamic Vinaigrette (recipe follows)
- 12 ounces tuna steaks
- 2 teaspoons Dijon mustard
- 8 ounces small shell pasta, cooked and drained
- 4 cups torn red leaf lettuce
- 2 cups sliced asparagus, cooked crisp-tender and cooled
- ½ cup thinly sliced fennel bulb
- ½ cup thinly sliced red bell pepper
- 8 cherry tomatoes, halved
- Salt and black pepper (optional)

1 Prepare grill for direct cooking over medium-high heat or preheat broiler. Prepare Balsamic Vinaigrette.

2 Brush sides of tuna with mustard. Grill tuna or broil 6 inches from heat source about 5 minutes per side or until fish begins to flake when tested with fork. Break into chunks.

3 Combine tuna, pasta, lettuce, asparagus, fennel, bell pepper and tomatoes in large bowl. Drizzle with Balsamic Vinaigrette; toss gently to coat. Season with salt and black pepper, if desired.

Balsamic Vinaigrette

Combine ¼ cup water, ¼ cup balsamic vinegar, 3 tablespoons olive oil, 2 tablespoons minced red onion, 3 cloves minced garlic, ¾ teaspoon dried chervil and ½ teaspoon celery seeds in small jar with tight-fitting lid; refrigerate until ready to use. Shake well before using.

Southwestern Chicken Salad

MAKES 6 SERVINGS

Salad

- 1 can (about 15 ounces) no-salt-added black beans, rinsed and drained
- 12 ounces cooked skinless chicken breast, cut into ½-inch pieces
- 1 can (8 ounces) diced water chestnuts
- ½ red bell pepper, seeded and diced
- ½ green bell pepper, seeded and diced
- ¼ red onion, chopped
- ½ cup chopped fresh cilantro
- ½ jalapeño pepper, minced (optional)

Dressing

- 3 tablespoons cider vinegar
- 2 tablespoons olive oil
- 2 tablespoons orange juice
- 1 teaspoon ground cumin
- ½ teaspoon chili powder
- ½ teaspoon ground red pepper
- ¼ teaspoon salt

1. Combine beans, chicken, water chestnuts, bell peppers, onion, cilantro and jalapeño in large bowl.
2. Combine vinegar, oil, orange juice, cumin, chili powder, ground red pepper and salt in small jar with tight-fitting lid; shake until well blended.
3. Pour dressing over salad; toss to coat.

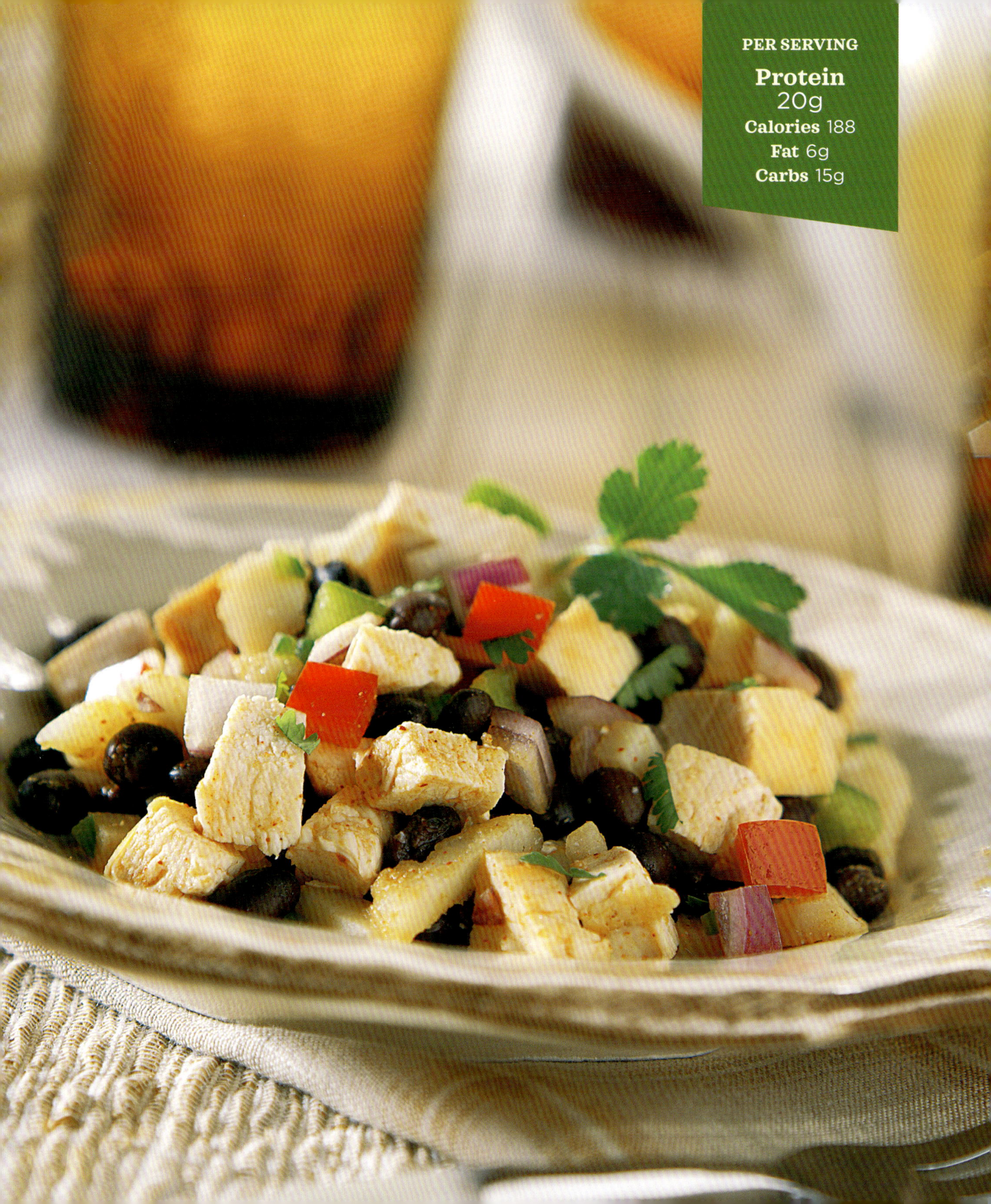
PER SERVING
Protein
20g
Calories 188
Fat 6g
Carbs 15g

PER SERVING
Protein
25g
Calories 240
Fat 7g
Carbs 21g

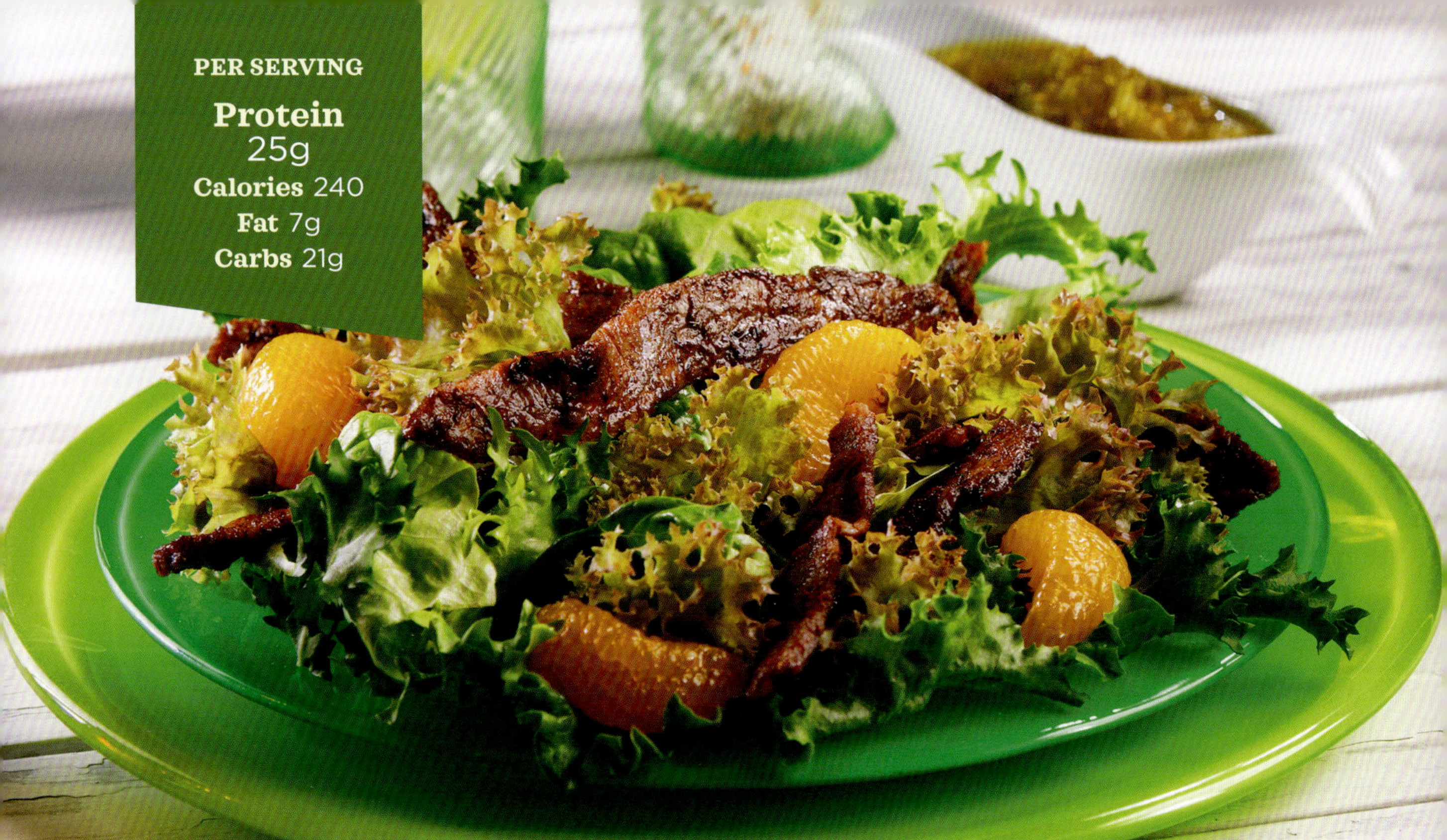

Tex-Mex Flank Steak Salad

MAKES 2 SERVINGS

- 8 ounces beef flank steak
- ½ teaspoon Mexican seasoning blend or chili powder
- ⅛ teaspoon salt
- 4 cups mixed greens
- 1 can (11 ounces) mandarin orange sections, drained
- 2 tablespoons green taco sauce

1. Cut steak in half lengthwise, then cut crosswise into thin strips. Combine Mexican seasoning and salt in medium bowl. Add steak; toss to coat.
2. Lightly spray large skillet with olive oil cooking spray; heat over medium-high heat. Add steak; cook and stir 1 to 2 minutes or until desired doneness.
3. Combine mixed greens and orange sections in large bowl; arrange on serving plates. Top with warm steak; drizzle with taco sauce.

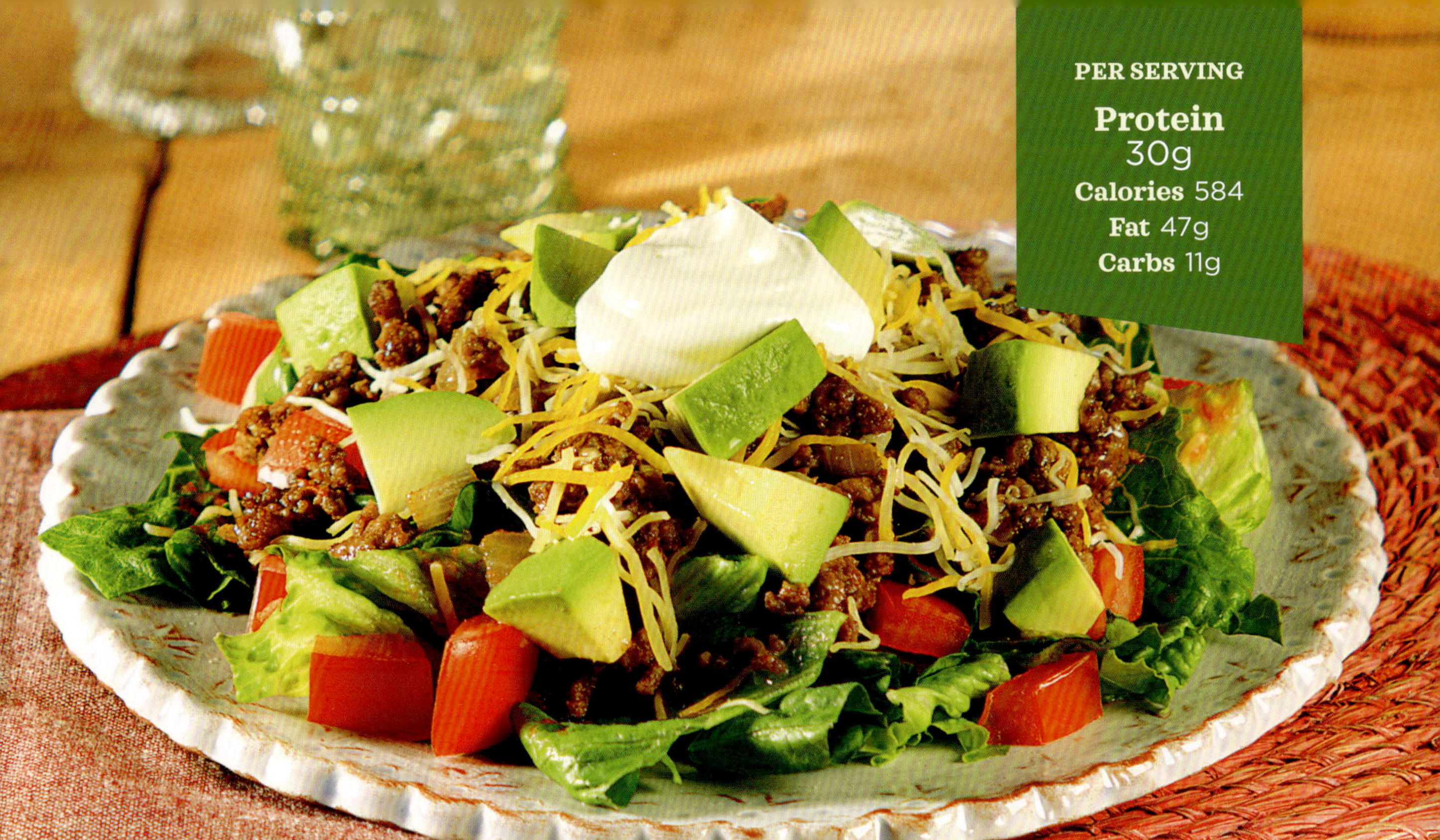

PER SERVING

Protein 30g

Calories 584

Fat 47g

Carbs 11g

Taco Salad Supreme

MAKES 4 SERVINGS

- 1 pound ground beef
- ½ cup chopped onion
- 2 cloves garlic, minced
- 1 teaspoon ground cumin
- 1 teaspoon chili powder
- ½ teaspoon salt
- ½ cup salsa, divided
- 6 cups packed torn or sliced romaine lettuce
- 1 large tomato, chopped
- 1 cup (4 ounces) shredded Mexican or taco cheese blend, divided
- 2 tablespoons canola oil
- 1 ripe avocado, diced
- ¼ cup sour cream

1. Cook beef and onion in large skillet over medium-high heat 6 to 8 minutes or until browned, stirring to break up meat. Drain fat.

2. Add garlic, cumin, chili powder and salt; cook and stir 1 minute. Add ¼ cup salsa; cook and stir 1 minute. Remove from heat.

3. Combine lettuce, tomato, ½ cup cheese, remaining ¼ cup salsa and oil in large bowl; mix gently.

4. Divide salad among four serving plates. Spoon meat mixture evenly over salads; top with remaining ½ cup cheese, avocado and sour cream.

Quinoa and Shrimp Salad

MAKES 4 TO 6 SERVINGS

- **1 cup uncooked quinoa**
- **2 cups water**
- **½ teaspoon salt, divided**
- **12 ounces thawed frozen cooked small shrimp, well drained**
- **1 cup cherry or grape tomatoes, halved**
- **¼ cup chopped fresh basil**
- **2 tablespoons capers**
- **2 tablespoons finely chopped green onion**
- **3 tablespoons olive oil**
- **1 to 2 tablespoons lemon juice**
- **1 teaspoon grated lemon peel**
- **⅛ teaspoon black pepper**

1. Place quinoa in fine-mesh strainer; rinse well under cold water. Bring 2 cups water and ¼ teaspoon salt to a boil in medium saucepan over high heat. Stir in quinoa. Reduce heat to low; cover and simmer 10 to 15 minutes or until quinoa is tender and water is absorbed.
2. Combine quinoa, shrimp, tomatoes, basil, capers and green onion in large bowl. Whisk oil, lemon juice, lemon peel, pepper and remaining ¼ teaspoon salt in small bowl until well blended.
3. Pour dressing over salad; toss gently to coat.

Tip

To avoid soggy shrimp, drain them well and blot dry on paper towels before adding them to the salad.

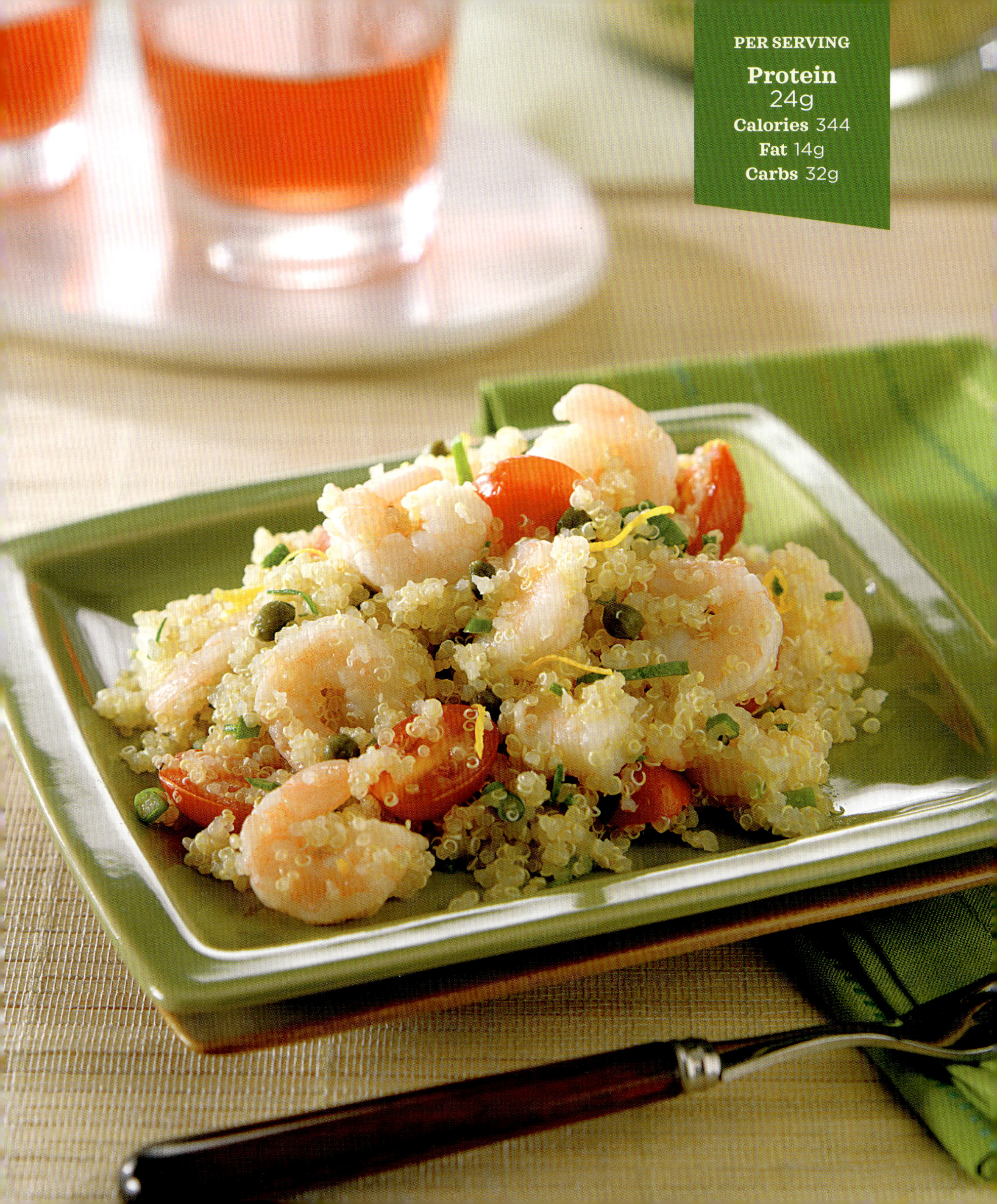
PER SERVING
Protein
24g
Calories 344
Fat 14g
Carbs 32g

Greek Lentil Salad with Feta Vinaigrette

MAKES 3 SERVINGS

- **4 cups water**
- **¾ cup dried lentils, rinsed and sorted**
- **1 bay leaf**
- **1 cup grape tomatoes, halved**
- **1 large stalk celery, chopped**
- **¼ cup chopped green onions**
- **¼ cup (1 ounce) crumbled feta cheese**
- **2 tablespoons olive oil**
- **1 tablespoon white wine vinegar**
- **½ teaspoon dried thyme**
- **½ teaspoon dried oregano**
- **½ teaspoon salt**
- **¼ teaspoon black pepper**

1. Combine water, lentils and bay leaf in small saucepan; bring to a boil over high heat. Reduce heat to medium-low; partially cover and cook 40 minutes or until lentils are tender but not mushy.

2. Drain lentils; remove and discard bay leaf. Place lentils in serving bowl; stir in tomatoes, celery and green onions.

3. Whisk cheese, oil, vinegar, thyme, oregano, salt and pepper in small bowl until well blended.

4. Pour dressing over salad; stir gently to coat. Let stand at least 10 minutes to allow flavors to blend.

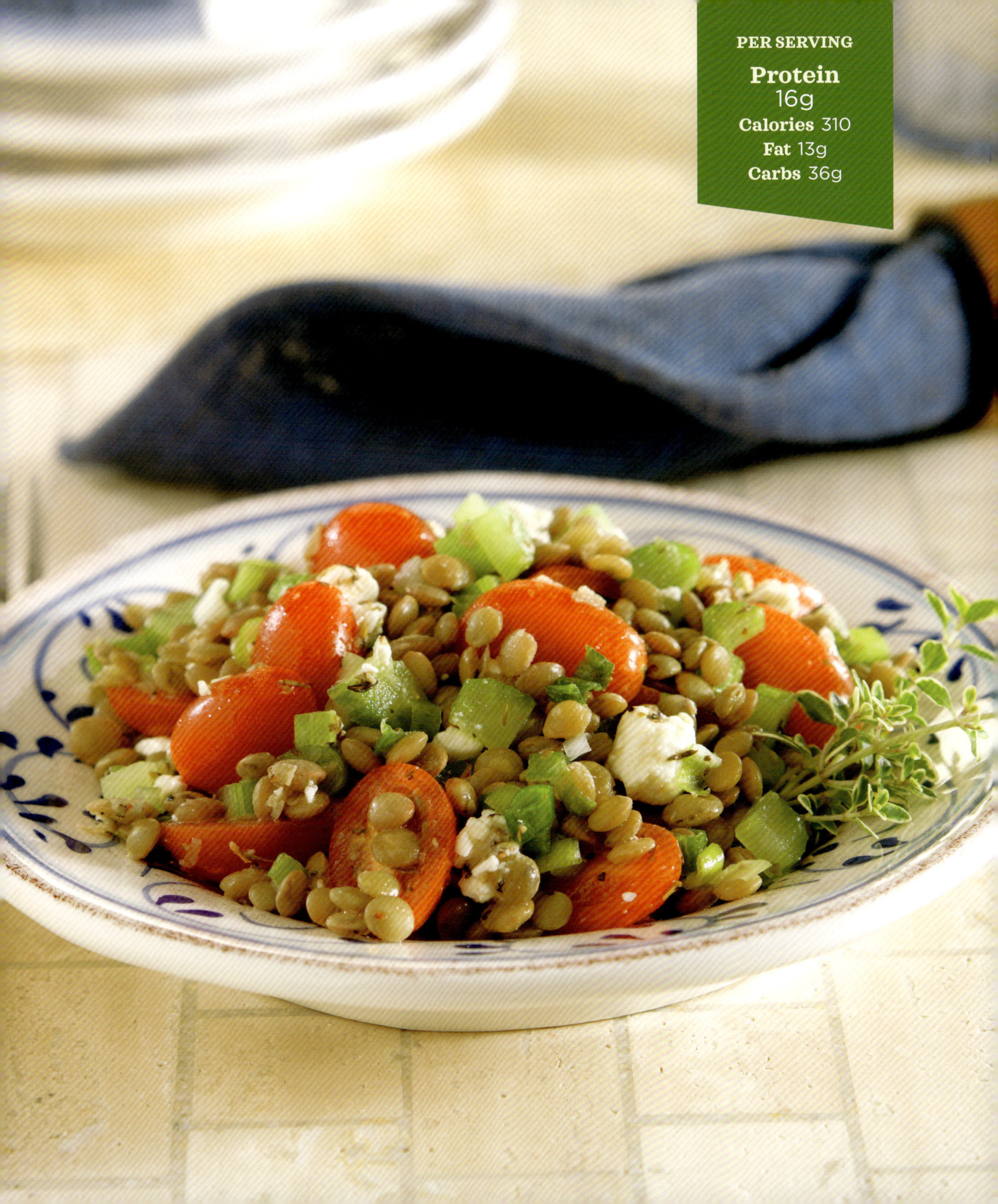
PER SERVING
Protein
16g
Calories 310
Fat 13g
Carbs 36g

Warm Salmon Salad

MAKES 4 SERVINGS

- Chive Vinaigrette (recipe follows)
- 2 cups water
- ¼ cup chopped onion
- 2 tablespoons red wine vinegar
- ¼ teaspoon black pepper
- 1¼ pounds small unpeeled red potatoes
- 1 pound salmon steaks
- 6 cups mixed greens
- 2 medium tomatoes, cut into wedges
- 16 pitted Kalamata olives, sliced

1 Prepare Chive Vinaigrette; refrigerate until ready to use.

2 Combine water, onion, vinegar and pepper in large saucepan; bring to a boil over medium-high heat. Add potatoes. Reduce heat to medium-low; cover and cook 10 minutes or until fork-tender. Transfer potatoes to cutting board with slotted spoon; cool slightly. Reserve cooking water in saucepan.

3 Cut potatoes into thick slices; place in medium bowl. Add ⅓ cup vinaigrette; toss to coat.

4 Add salmon to reserved cooking water in saucepan; bring to a simmer over medium-low heat. Simmer gently 4 to 5 minutes or until fish is opaque and begins to flake when tested with fork. (Do not boil.) Remove salmon to cutting board; let stand 5 minutes. Remove and discard skin and bones; cut salmon into 1-inch pieces.

5 Divide mixed greens among four plates; top with salmon, potatoes, tomatoes and olives. Drizzle with remaining vinaigrette.

Chive Vinaigrette

Combine ⅓ cup vegetable oil, ¼ cup red wine vinegar, 2 tablespoons finely chopped fresh chives, 2 tablespoons finely chopped fresh parsley, ⅛ teaspoon salt and ⅛ teaspoon white pepper in small jar with tight-fitting lid; shake until well blended.

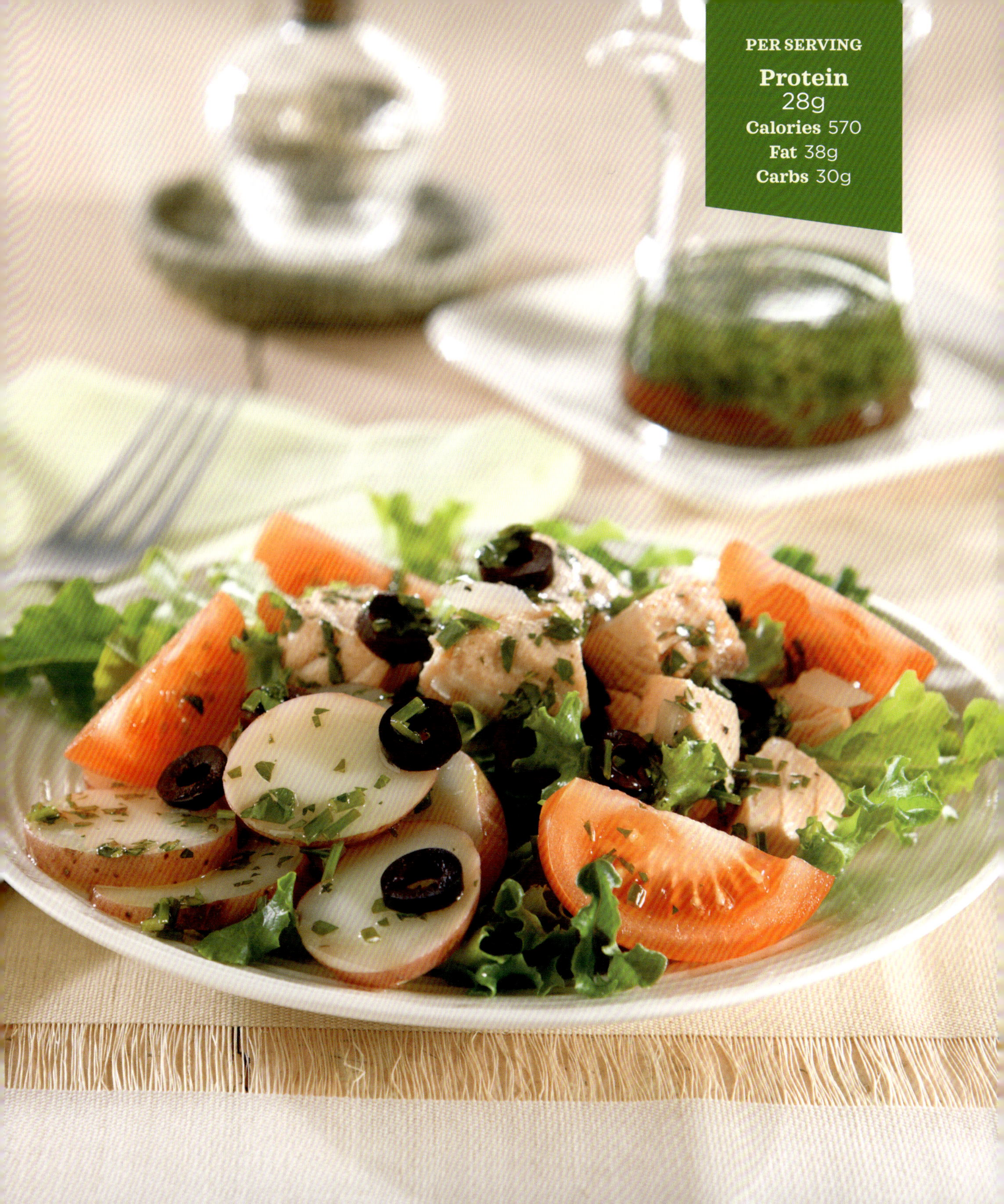
PER SERVING
Protein
28g
Calories 570
Fat 38g
Carbs 30g

Thai Chicken Broccoli Salad

MAKES 4 SERVINGS

- 4 ounces uncooked linguine
- 8 ounces boneless skinless chicken breasts, cut into bite-size pieces
- 2 cups broccoli florets
- 2 tablespoons cold water
- ⅔ cup chopped red bell pepper
- 6 green onions, cut diagonally into 1-inch pieces
- ¼ cup reduced-fat creamy peanut butter
- 2 tablespoons hot water
- 2 tablespoons reduced-sodium soy sauce
- 2 teaspoons dark sesame oil
- ½ teaspoon red pepper flakes
- ⅛ teaspoon garlic powder
- ¼ cup unsalted peanuts, chopped

1. Cook pasta according to package directions, omitting salt. Drain.
2. Spray large nonstick skillet with cooking spray; heat over medium-high heat. Add chicken; cook and stir 5 minutes or until chicken is cooked through. Transfer to large bowl.
3. Add broccoli and cold water to skillet; cover and cook 2 minutes over medium-high heat. Uncover; cook and stir 2 minutes or until broccoli is crisp-tender. Transfer broccoli to bowl with chicken; add pasta, bell pepper and green onions.
4. Whisk peanut butter, hot water, soy sauce, oil, red pepper flakes and garlic powder in small bowl until well blended.
5. Drizzle dressing over salad; toss to coat. Top with peanuts just before serving.

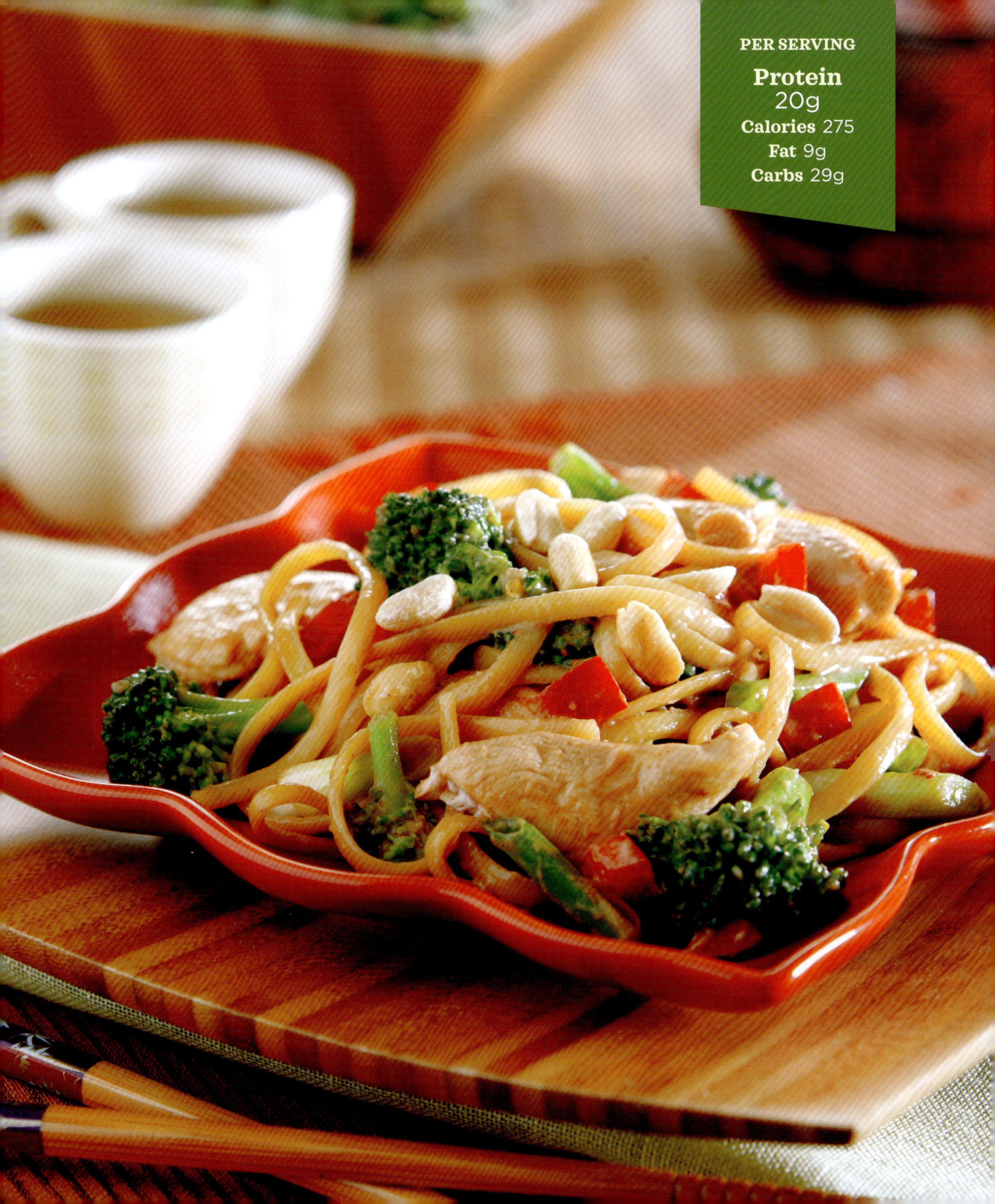
PER SERVING
Protein
20g
Calories 275
Fat 9g
Carbs 29g

Crab Spinach Salad with Tarragon Dressing

MAKES 4 SERVINGS

- 12 ounces coarsely flaked cooked crabmeat *or* 2 packages (6 ounces each) frozen crabmeat, thawed and drained
- 1 cup chopped tomatoes
- 1 cup sliced cucumber
- ⅓ cup sliced red onion
- ¼ cup fat-free salad dressing or mayonnaise
- ¼ cup reduced-fat sour cream
- ¼ cup chopped fresh parsley
- 2 tablespoons fat-free (skim) milk
- 2 teaspoons chopped fresh tarragon *or* ½ teaspoon dried tarragon leaves
- 1 clove garlic, minced
- ¼ teaspoon hot pepper sauce
- 8 cups fresh spinach

1. Combine crabmeat, tomatoes, cucumber and onion in medium bowl. Whisk salad dressing, sour cream, parsley, milk, tarragon, garlic and hot pepper sauce in small bowl until well blended.

2. Line four plates with spinach. Top with crabmeat mixture; drizzle with dressing.

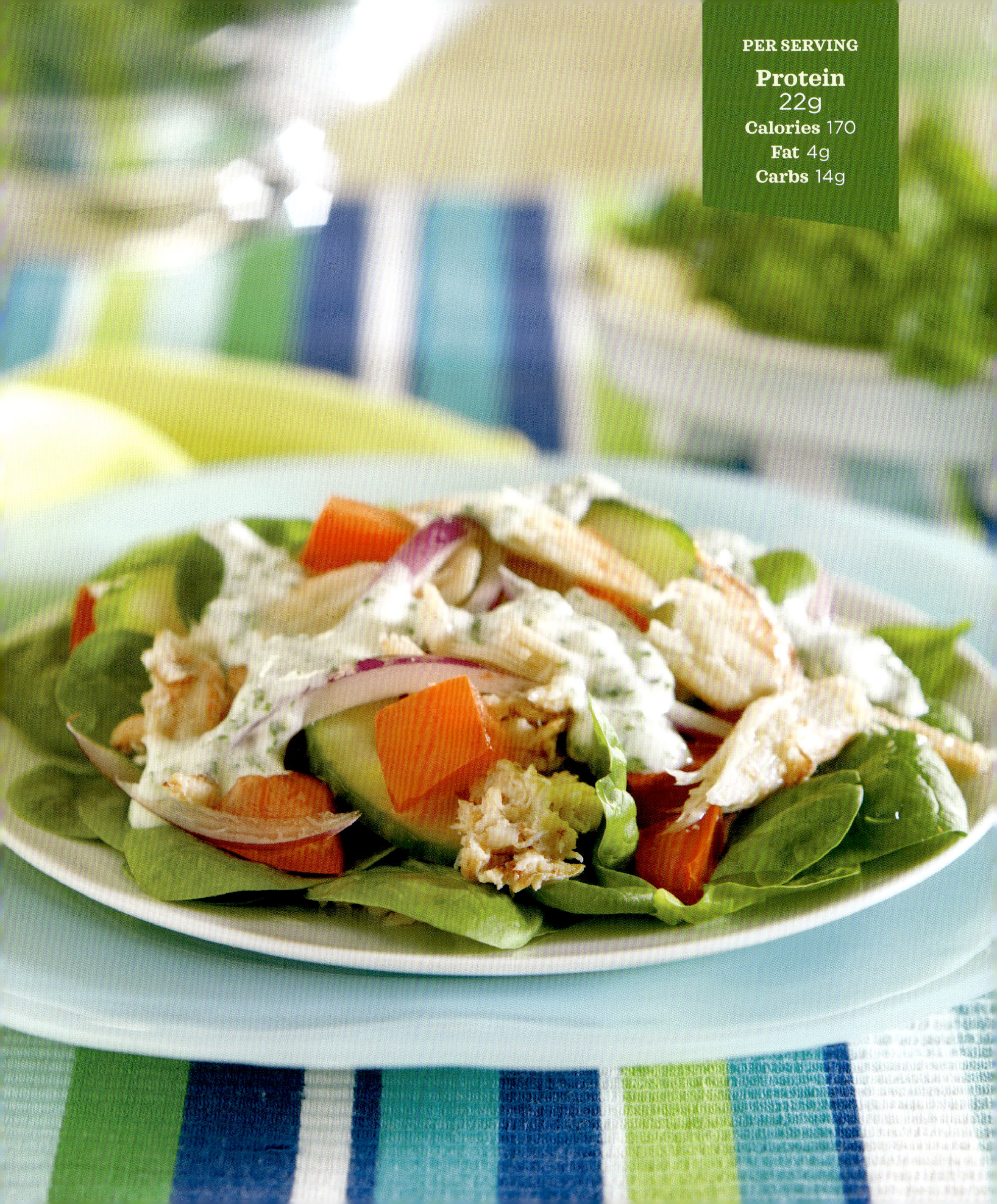
PER SERVING
Protein
22g
Calories 170
Fat 4g
Carbs 14g

Mixed Greens with Pear and Goat Cheese

MAKES 4 SERVINGS

Dressing

- ¼ cup balsamic vinegar
- 1½ tablespoons olive oil
- 2 tablespoons honey
- 1 small clove garlic, minced
- ½ teaspoon salt
- ¼ teaspoon black pepper

Salad

- 1 package (5 ounces) spring greens salad blend
- 2 pears, thinly sliced
- 1 cup chopped cooked chicken (about 5 ounces)
- ½ cup chopped celery
- ⅓ cup crumbled goat cheese
- 2 tablespoons slivered almonds (optional)

1 Whisk vinegar, oil, honey, garlic, salt and pepper in small bowl until well blended.

2 Combine greens, pears, chicken, celery and cheese in large bowl. Drizzle dressing over salad; toss gently to coat. Top with almonds, if desired.

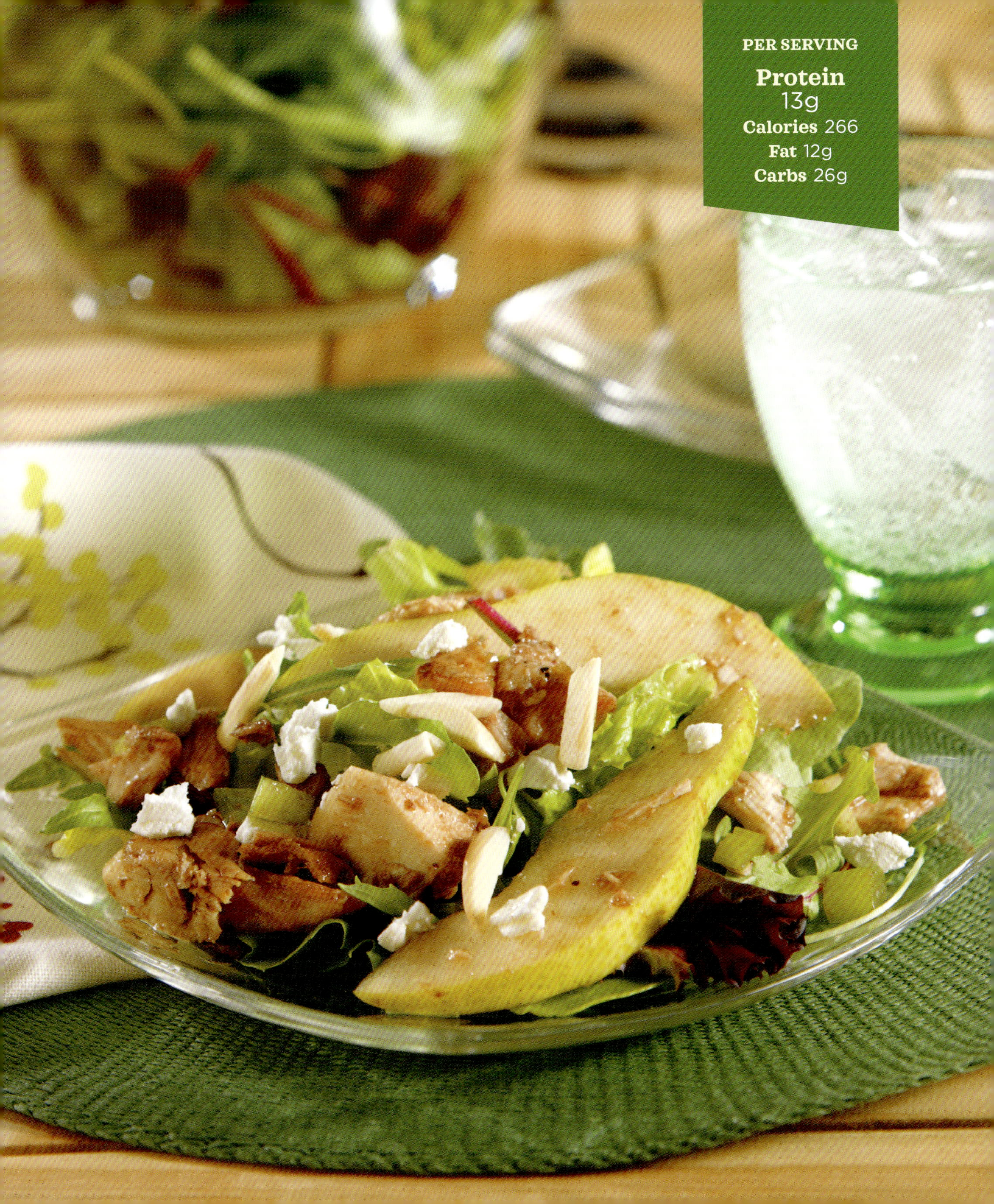
PER SERVING
Protein
13g
Calories 266
Fat 12g
Carbs 26g

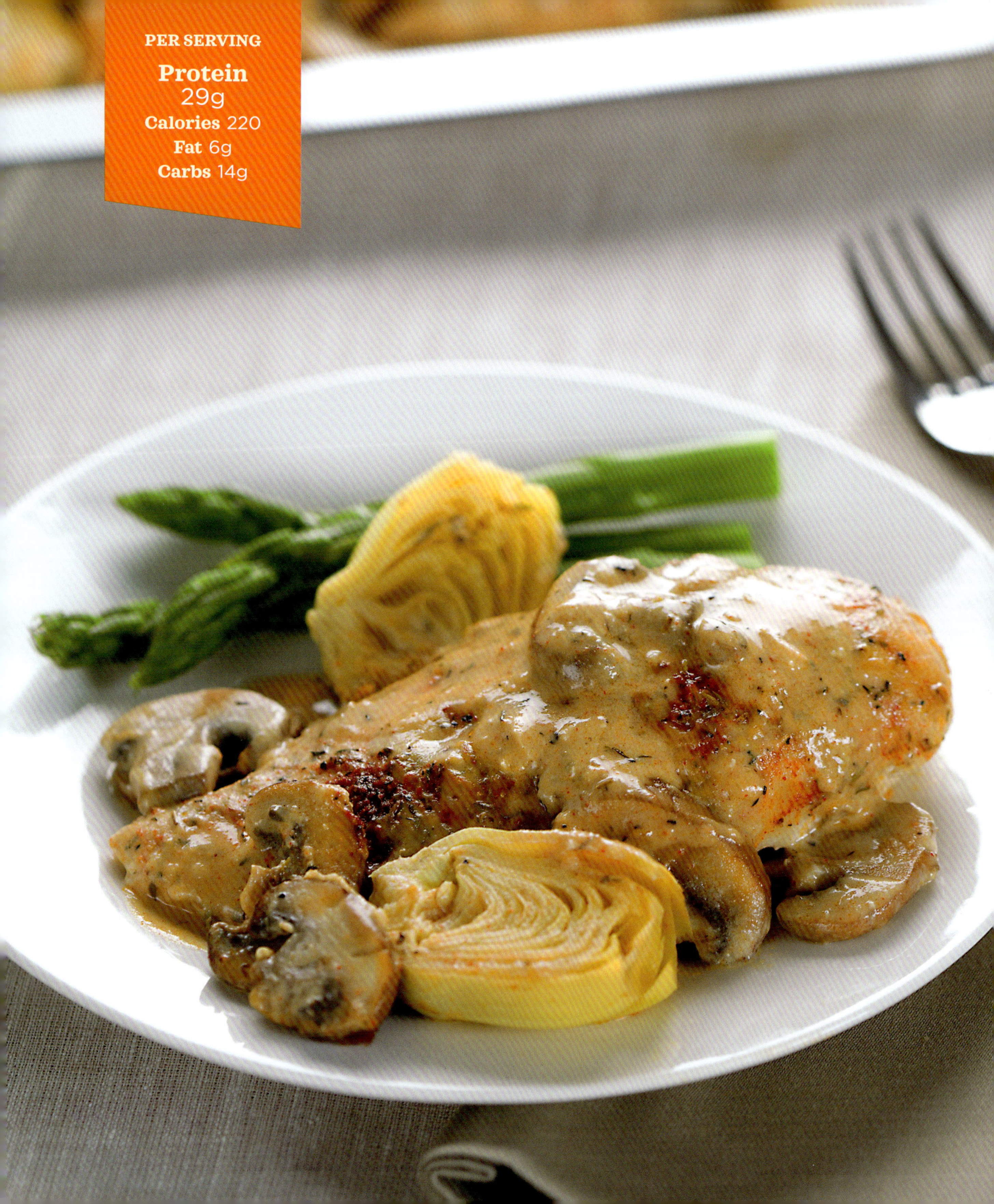
PER SERVING
Protein
29g
Calories 220
Fat 6g
Carbs 14g

POULTRY

Creamy Baked Chicken with Artichokes and Mushrooms

MAKES 6 SERVINGS

- 6 boneless skinless chicken breasts (4 to 6 ounces each)
- 1½ teaspoons paprika
- 1½ teaspoons dried thyme
- ½ teaspoon salt
- ½ teaspoon black pepper
- 1 can (14 ounces) artichokes packed in water, drained
- 1 tablespoon butter
- 1 package (8 ounces) sliced cremini mushrooms
- 2 tablespoons all-purpose flour
- ¾ cup reduced-sodium chicken broth
- ½ cup half-and-half

1. Preheat oven to 375°F.

2. Place chicken in 13×9-inch baking dish. Combine paprika, thyme, salt and pepper in small bowl; mix well. Reserve 1 teaspoon spice mixture for sauce; sprinkle remaining spice mixture evenly over chicken. Cut artichokes in half; arrange around chicken.

3. Melt butter in large saucepan over medium heat. Add mushrooms and reserved 1 teaspoon spice mixture; cook and stir 5 minutes or until tender. Sprinkle flour over mushrooms; cook and stir 1 minute. Stir in broth; cook 3 minutes or until thickened. Stir in half-and-half; cook 1 minute. Pour over chicken and artichokes.

4. Bake 30 minutes or until chicken is no longer pink in center (165°F).

Greek Chicken Burgers with Cucumber Yogurt Sauce

MAKES 4 SERVINGS

- ½ cup plus 2 tablespoons plain nonfat Greek yogurt
- ½ medium cucumber, peeled, seeded and finely chopped
- Juice of ½ lemon
- 3 cloves garlic, minced, divided
- 2 teaspoons finely chopped fresh mint *or* ½ teaspoon dried mint
- ⅛ teaspoon salt
- ⅛ teaspoon ground white pepper
- 1 pound ground chicken
- ¾ cup (3 ounces) crumbled reduced-fat feta cheese
- 4 large Kalamata olives, rinsed, patted dry and minced
- 1 egg
- ½ to 1 teaspoon dried oregano
- ¼ teaspoon black pepper
- Mixed greens (optional)
- Fresh mint leaves (optional)

1 Combine yogurt, cucumber, lemon juice, 2 cloves garlic, 2 teaspoons chopped mint, salt and white pepper in medium bowl; mix well. Cover and refrigerate until ready to serve.

2 Combine chicken, cheese, olives, egg, oregano, black pepper and remaining 1 clove garlic in large bowl; mix gently. Shape mixture into four patties.

3 Spray grill pan with nonstick cooking spray; heat over medium-high heat. Grill patties 5 to 7 minutes per side or until cooked through (165°F).

4 Serve burgers with sauce and mixed greens, if desired. Garnish with mint leaves.

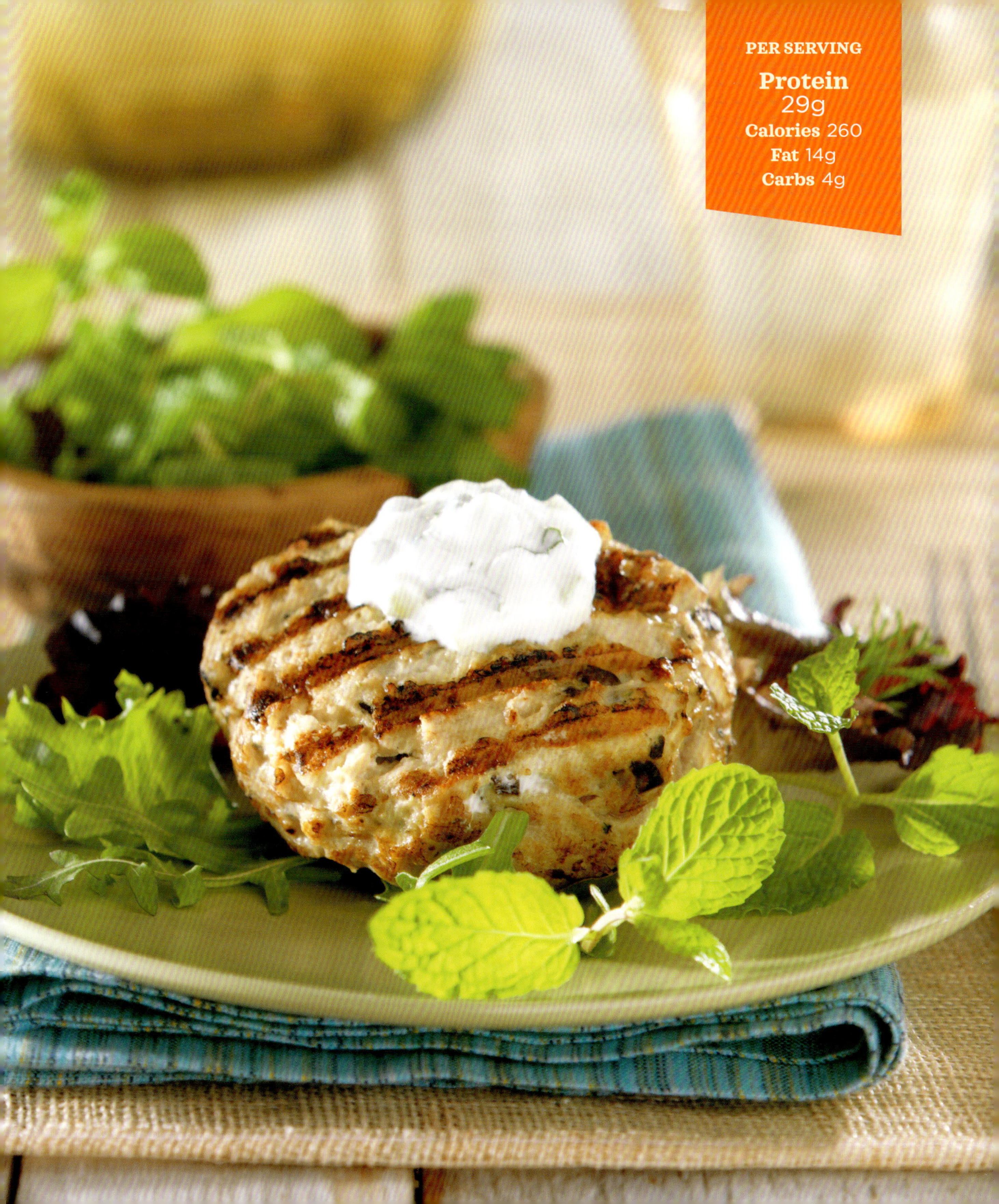
PER SERVING
Protein
29g
Calories 260
Fat 14g
Carbs 4g

Turkey Vegetable Meatballs

MAKES 6 SERVINGS

- **1 pound lean ground turkey**
- **½ cup finely chopped green onions**
- **½ cup finely chopped green bell pepper**
- **⅓ cup old-fashioned oats**
- **¼ cup shredded carrot**
- **¼ cup grated Parmesan cheese**
- **2 egg whites**
- **2 tablespoons whipping cream**
- **2 cloves garlic, minced**
- **½ teaspoon Italian seasoning**
- **¼ teaspoon fennel seeds**
- **¼ teaspoon salt**
- **⅛ teaspoon red pepper flakes (optional)**
- **1 teaspoon olive oil**

1 Combine turkey, green onions, bell pepper, oats, carrot, cheese, egg whites, cream, garlic, Italian seasoning, fennel seeds, salt and red pepper flakes, if desired, in large bowl; mix gently. Shape into 36 (1-inch) balls.

2 Heat oil in large nonstick skillet over medium-high heat. Add meatballs; cook 11 minutes or until cooked through (165°F), turning frequently. (Use fork and spoon for easy turning.) Serve immediately or cool and freeze.*

**To freeze, cool completely and place in gallon-size resealable food storage bag. Release any excess air from bag and seal. Freeze bag flat for easier storage and faster thawing. This will also allow you to remove as many meatballs as needed without them sticking together. To reheat, place meatballs in a 12×8-inch microwavable dish and cook on HIGH 20 to 30 seconds or until hot.*

Serving Suggestion

Top meatballs with a meatless marinara sauce.

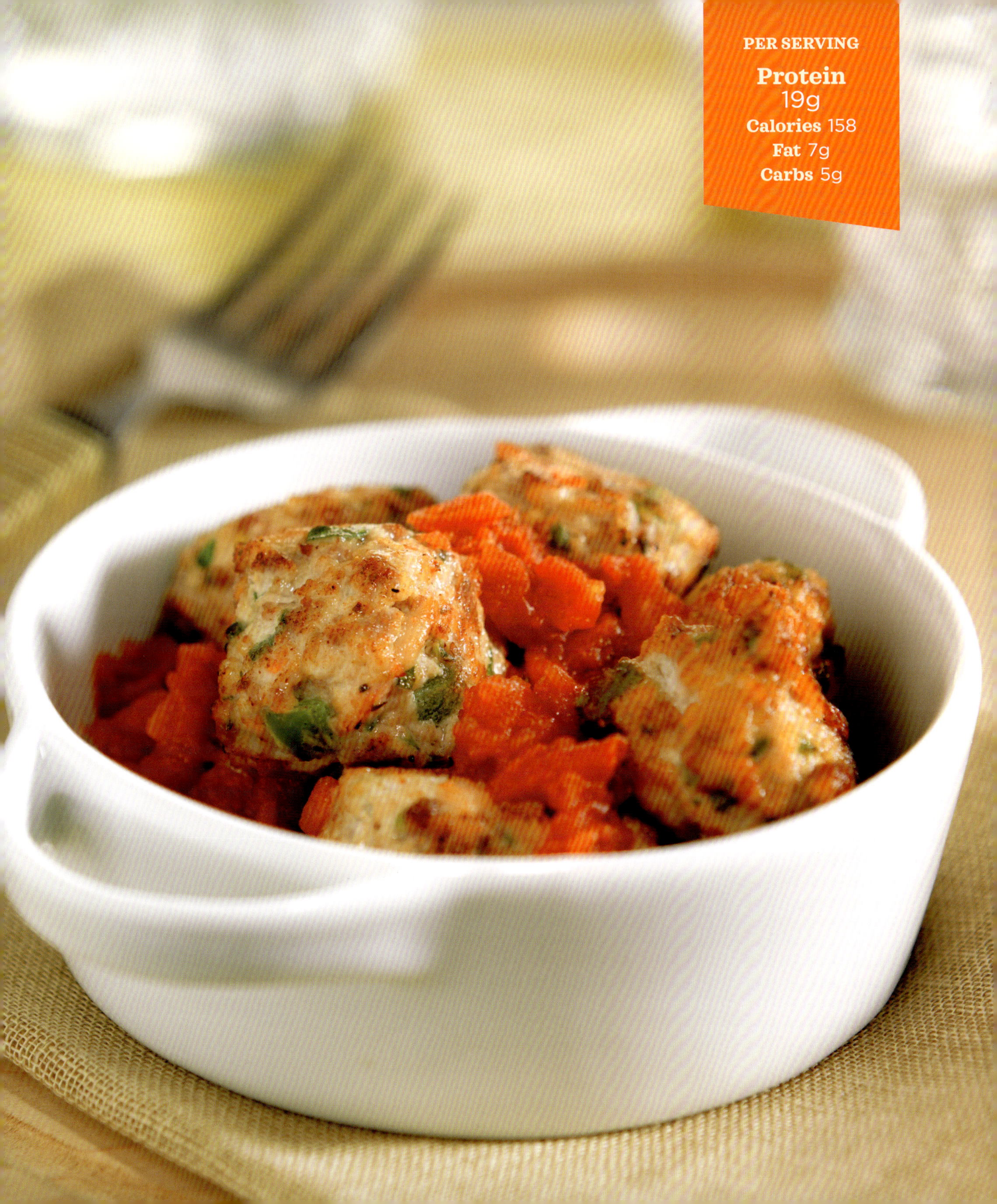
PER SERVING
Protein
19g
Calories 158
Fat 7g
Carbs 5g

Kale and Mushroom Stuffed Chicken Breasts

MAKES 4 SERVINGS

- **3 teaspoons olive oil, divided**
- **1 cup coarsely chopped mushrooms**
- **2 cups thinly sliced kale**
- **1 tablespoon lemon juice**
- **½ teaspoon salt, divided**
- **4 boneless skinless chicken breasts (about 4 ounces each)**
- **¼ cup (1 ounce) crumbled fat-free feta cheese**
- **¼ teaspoon black pepper**

1 Heat 1 teaspoon oil in large skillet over medium-high heat. Add mushrooms; cook and stir 5 minutes or until mushrooms begin to brown. Add kale; cook and stir 8 minutes or until wilted. Stir in lemon juice and ¼ teaspoon salt. Remove to small bowl; let stand 5 to 10 minutes to cool slightly.

2 Meanwhile, place chicken between two sheets of plastic wrap; pound to ½-inch thickness with meat mallet or rolling pin.

3 Gently stir cheese into kale mixture. Spoon ¼ cup mixture down center of each chicken breast. Roll up chicken to enclose filling; secure with toothpicks. Sprinkle with remaining ¼ teaspoon salt and pepper.

4 Wipe out same skillet with paper towels. Add remaining 2 teaspoons oil to skillet; heat over medium heat. Add chicken; cook until browned on all sides. Cover and cook 5 minutes per side or until no longer pink (165°F). Remove toothpicks before serving.

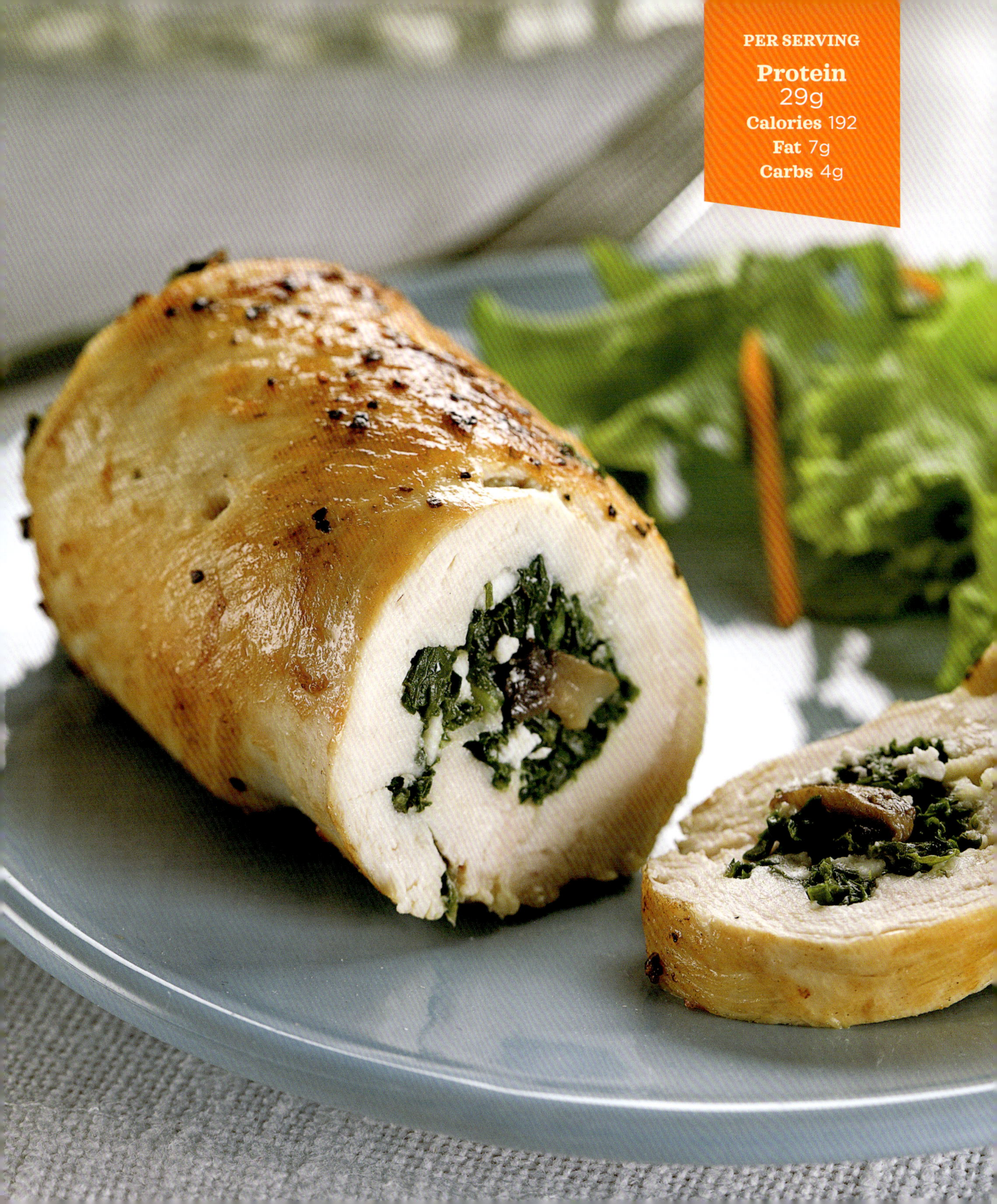
PER SERVING
Protein
29g
Calories 192
Fat 7g
Carbs 4g

PER SERVING
Protein
42g
Calories 360
Fat 18g
Carbs 5g

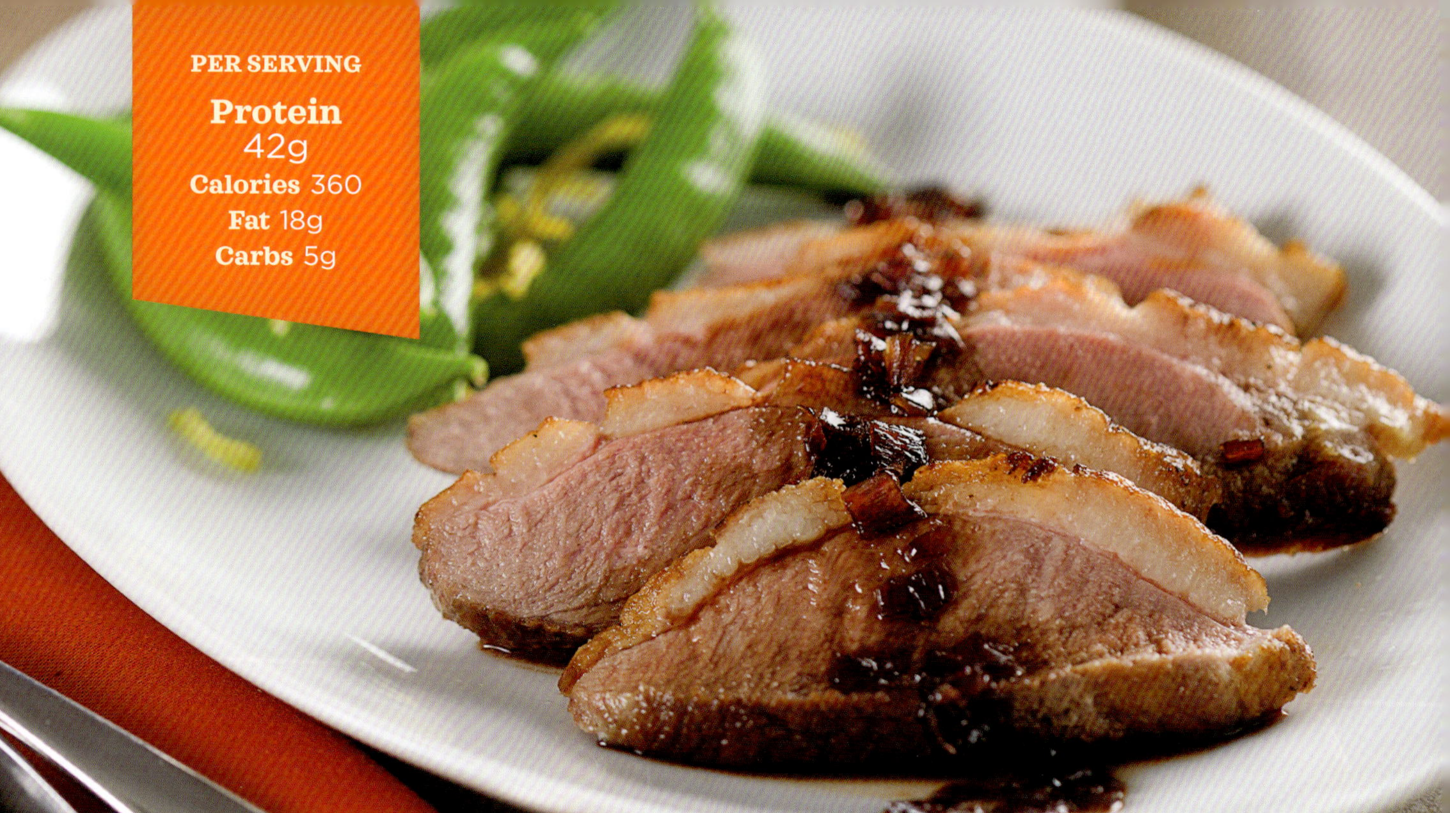

Duck Breasts with Balsamic Sauce

MAKES 4 SERVINGS

- **3 tablespoons balsamic vinegar**
- **2 tablespoons lemon juice**
- **4 boneless duck breasts (6 ounces each)**
- **Salt and black pepper**
- **1 shallot, minced**

1. Combine vinegar and lemon juice in small bowl.
2. Score skin on duck breasts with tip of sharp knife in crosshatch pattern, being careful to cut only into the fat and not the meat. Season both sides of duck with salt and pepper.
3. Place duck breasts skin side down in large skillet over medium heat; cook without turning 10 to 12 minutes or until skin is crisp and golden brown. Turn and cook about 8 minutes or until medium rare (130°F). Remove duck to plate; tent with foil and let stand 10 minutes before slicing.
4. Meanwhile, drain all but 1 tablespoon fat from skillet. Add shallot to skillet; cook and stir over medium heat 2 to 3 minutes or until translucent. Add vinegar mixture; cook and stir about 5 minutes or until slightly reduced. Season with salt and pepper. Slice duck; drizzle with sauce.

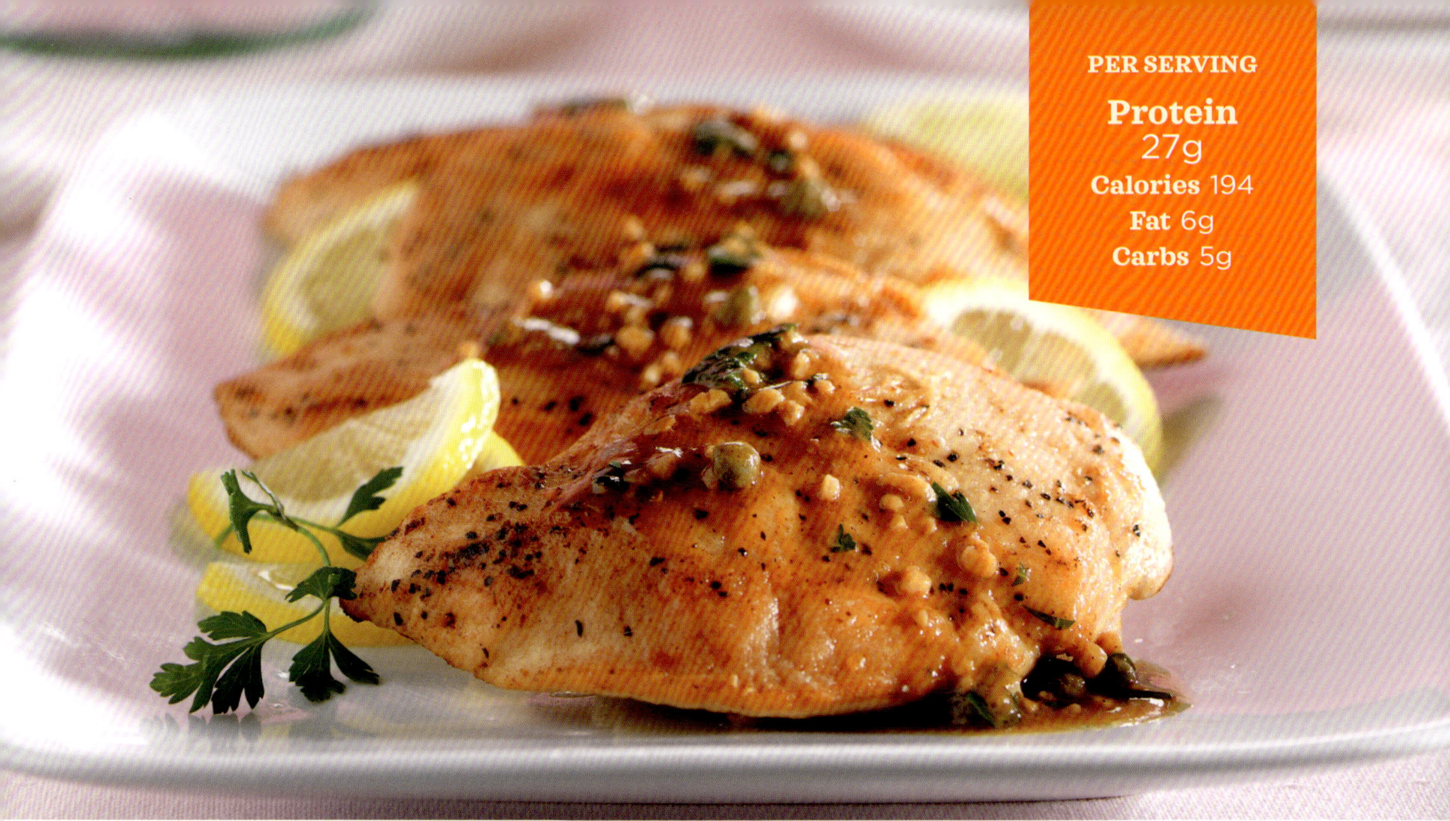

PER SERVING
Protein 27g
Calories 194
Fat 6g
Carbs 5g

Chicken Piccata

MAKES 4 SERVINGS

- **3 tablespoons all-purpose flour**
- **½ teaspoon salt**
- **¼ teaspoon black pepper**
- **4 boneless skinless chicken breasts (4 ounces each)**
- **2 teaspoons olive oil**
- **1 teaspoon butter**
- **2 cloves garlic, minced**
- **¾ cup reduced-sodium chicken broth**
- **1 tablespoon lemon juice**
- **2 tablespoons chopped fresh Italian parsley**
- **1 tablespoon capers, drained**

1. Combine flour, salt and pepper in shallow dish. Reserve 1 tablespoon flour mixture for sauce.
2. Pound chicken to ½-inch thickness between sheets of waxed paper with meat mallet or rolling pin. Coat chicken with remaining flour mixture, shaking off excess.
3. Heat oil and butter in large nonstick skillet over medium heat. Add chicken; cook 4 to 5 minutes per side or until no longer pink in center (165°F). Remove to platter; tent with foil to keep warm.
4. Add garlic to skillet; cook and stir 1 minute. Add reserved flour mixture; cook and stir 1 minute. Add broth and lemon juice; cook 2 minutes or until sauce thickens, stirring frequently. Stir in parsley and capers; spoon sauce over chicken.

Roasted Chicken with Cabbage

MAKES 4 SERVINGS

- ⅓ cup olive oil, plus additional for pan
- 2 tablespoons red wine vinegar
- 2 cloves garlic, minced
- 1 teaspoon salt
- 1 teaspoon onion powder
- ¼ teaspoon paprika
- ¼ teaspoon black pepper
- 8 bone-in, skin-on chicken thighs (about 3 pounds)
- 2 medium onions, cut into ½-inch slices (do not separate into rings)
- 1 small head green cabbage (about 1½ pounds)
- Chopped fresh parsley (optional)

1. Preheat oven to 425°F. Brush baking sheet with oil.

2. Whisk ⅓ cup oil, vinegar, garlic, salt, onion powder, paprika and pepper in large bowl until well blended. Remove half of mixture to medium bowl; add chicken and turn to coat.

3. Add onion slices to large bowl with oil mixture; turn to coat. Arrange in single layer on prepared baking sheet. Cut cabbage in half through core (do not remove core). Cut each half into 1-inch wedges. Add cabbage to large bowl with oil mixture; turn to coat. Arrange cabbage over onions on baking sheet. Place chicken, skin side up, on top of cabbage.

4. Roast 50 to 55 minutes or until chicken is cooked through (165°F). Remove chicken to plate; tent with foil to keep warm.

5. Carefully drain liquid from baking sheet. Stir vegetables; roast 10 to 15 minutes or until edges begin to brown and cabbage is crisp-tender. Serve chicken with vegetables; garnish with parsley.

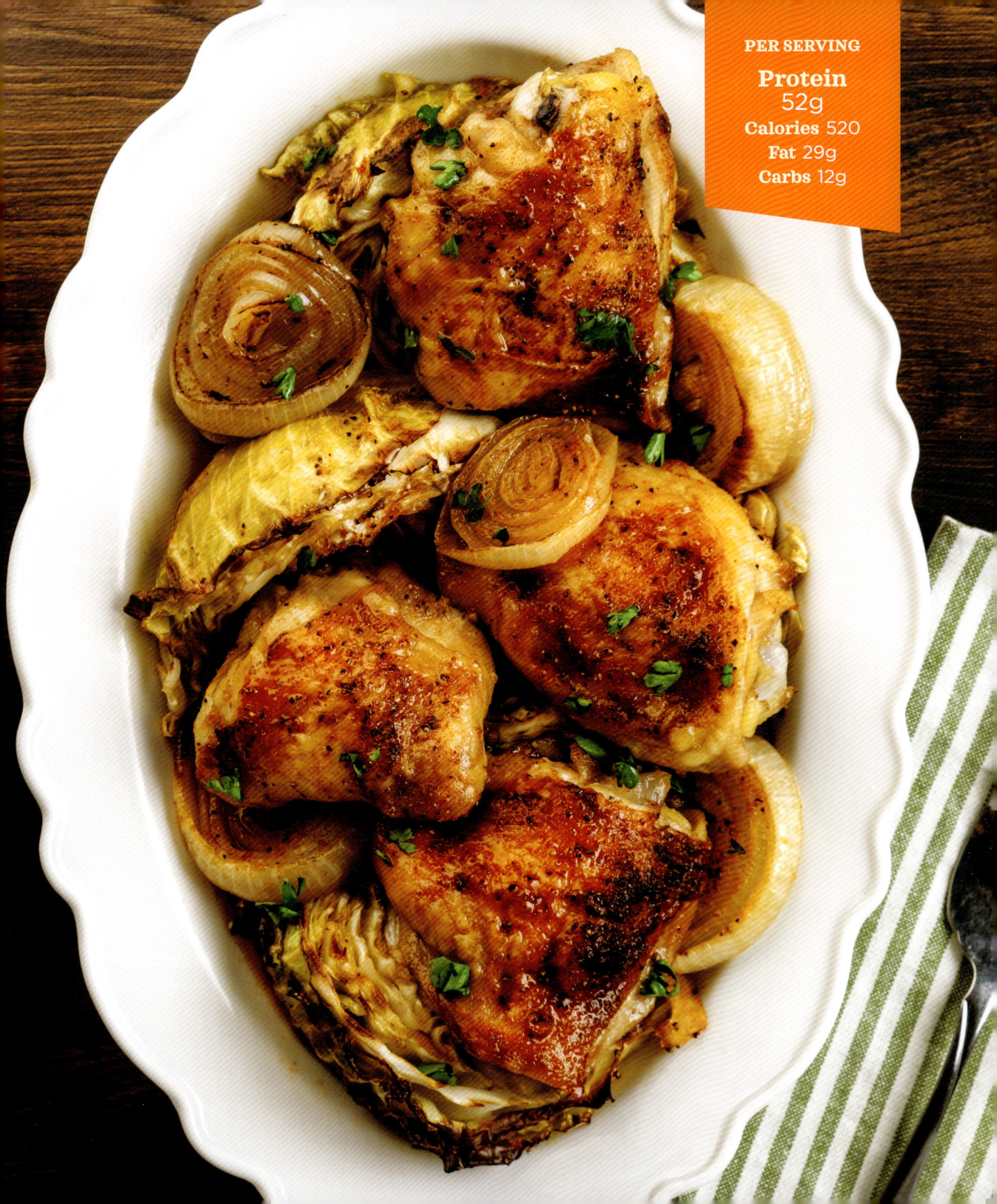
PER SERVING
Protein
52g
Calories 520
Fat 29g
Carbs 12g

Turkey Breast with Spinach-Blue Cheese Stuffing

MAKES 14 SERVINGS

- **1 frozen whole boneless turkey breast, thawed (3½ to 4 pounds)**
- **1 package (10 ounces) frozen chopped spinach, thawed and squeezed dry**
- **2 ounces blue cheese or feta cheese**
- **2 ounces reduced-fat cream cheese (Neufchâtel), softened**
- **½ cup finely chopped green onions**
- **1½ tablespoons Dijon mustard**
- **1½ tablespoons dried basil**
- **2 teaspoons dried oregano**
- **Salt, black pepper and paprika**

1. Preheat oven to 350°F. Spray roasting pan and rack with nonstick cooking spray.

2. Unroll turkey breast; pat dry. Place turkey between two sheets of plastic wrap or waxed paper; pound to 1-inch thickness with meat mallet or rolling pin. Remove and discard skin from one half of turkey breast; turn meat over so skin side on other half faces down.

3. Combine spinach, blue cheese, cream cheese, green onions, mustard, basil and oregano in medium bowl; mix well. Spread evenly over turkey breast. Roll up turkey so skin is on top. Tie closed with kitchen string.

4. Place turkey breast on prepared rack; season with salt, pepper and paprika. Roast 1½ hours or until no longer pink in center (165°F). Remove to cutting board; tent with foil and let stand 10 minutes. Remove skin; cut into ¼-inch-thick slices.

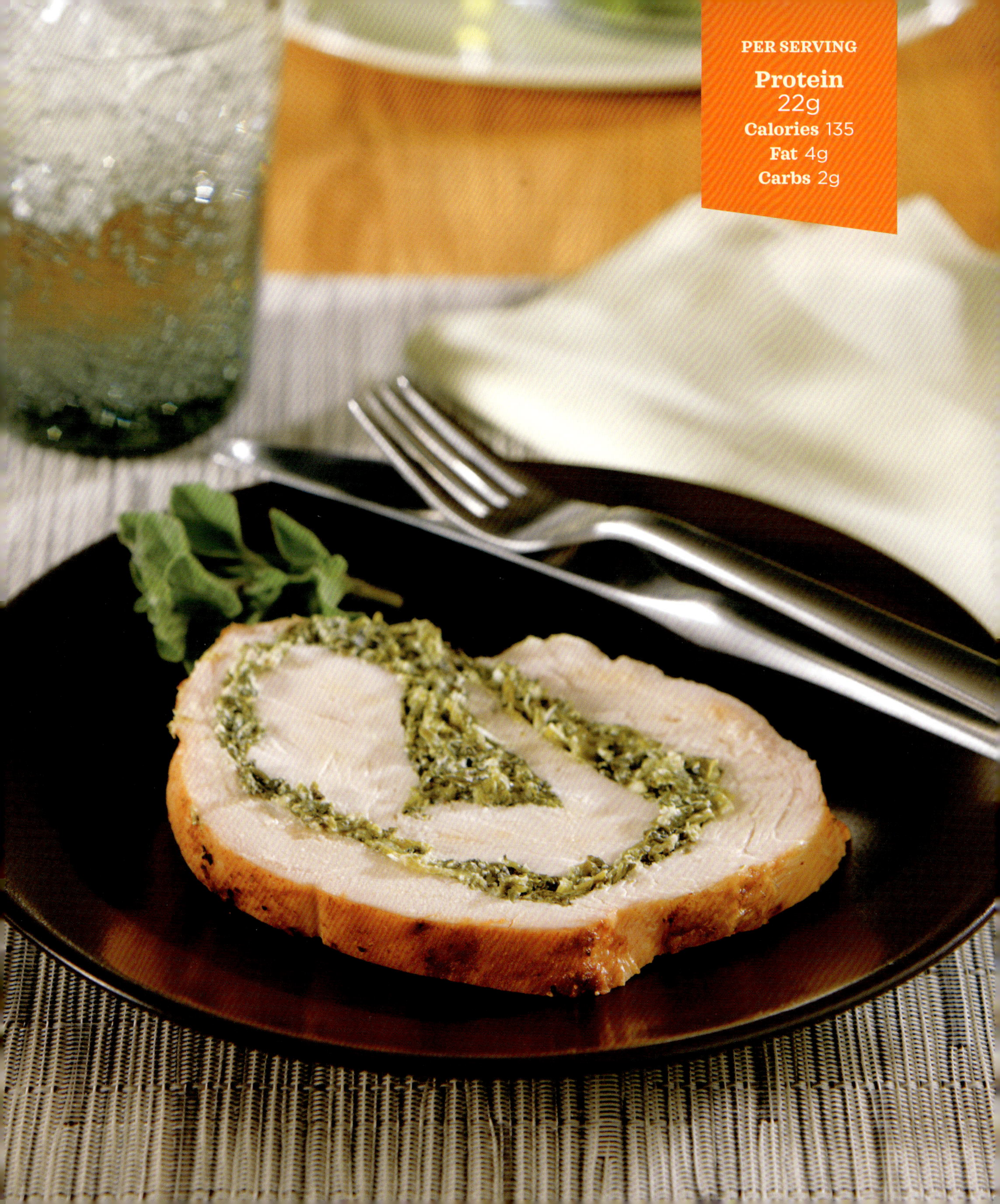
PER SERVING
Protein
22g
Calories 135
Fat 4g
Carbs 2g

Spatchcock Chicken and Vegetables

MAKES 4 SERVINGS

- 1 whole chicken (about 4 pounds)
- 6 tablespoons (¾ stick) butter, softened
- 2 tablespoons fresh thyme leaves
- 1 tablespoon honey
- 1 tablespoon Dijon mustard
- 1¼ teaspoons salt
- ½ teaspoon black pepper
- 12 ounces unpeeled small red potatoes, halved (about 12 (2-inch) potatoes)
- 8 ounces parsnips, cut diagonally into 1½-inch pieces (cut in half lengthwise if very thick)
- 8 ounces carrots, cut diagonally into 1½-inch pieces

1 Position oven rack in lower third of oven. Preheat oven to 425°F. Line baking sheet with foil, if desired.

2 To spatchcock chicken, place breast side down on cutting board. Cut along both sides of backbone with poultry shears or kitchen scissors; remove and discard backbone. Turn chicken breast side up; press down firmly on breast until it cracks to flatten chicken. Place on prepared baking sheet.

3 Combine butter, thyme, honey, mustard, salt and pepper in small microwavable bowl; mix well. Rub 1 tablespoon mixture under skin of chicken breast. Rub 1 tablespoon mixture all over chicken skin.

4 Combine potatoes, parsnips and carrots in large bowl. Melt remaining butter mixture in microwave; pour over vegetables and toss to coat. Arrange vegetables around chicken on baking sheet.

5 Roast 50 to 60 minutes or until chicken is cooked through (165°F), covering loosely with foil after 30 minutes if skin is turning too dark. Remove chicken to clean cutting board; tent with foil and let stand 10 minutes before slicing. Serve with vegetables.

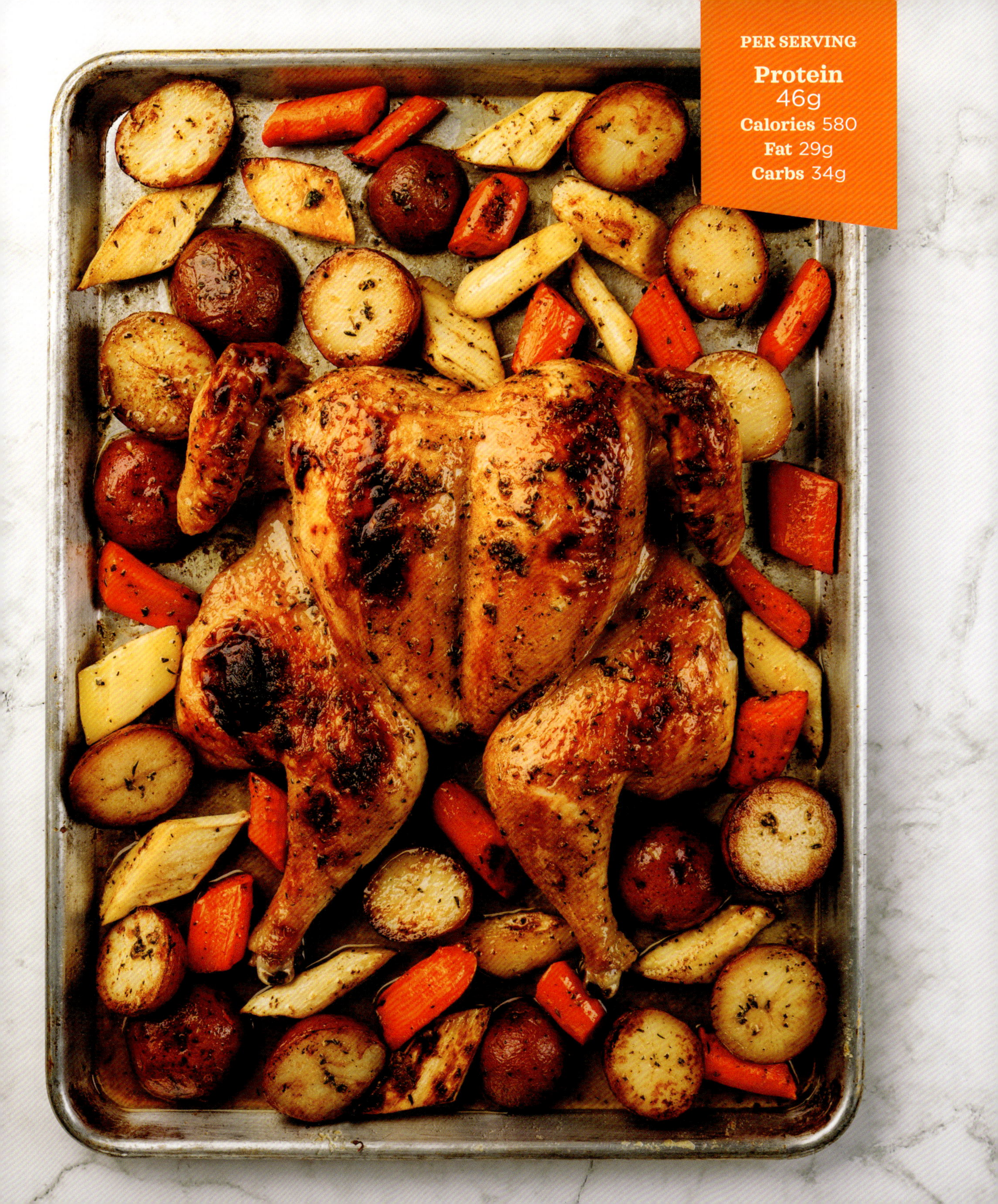
PER SERVING
Protein 46g
Calories 580
Fat 29g
Carbs 34g

Grilled Chicken with Chimichurri Salsa

MAKES 4 SERVINGS

- **4 boneless skinless chicken breasts (6 ounces each)**
- **½ cup plus 4 teaspoons olive oil, divided**
- **Salt and black pepper**
- **½ cup finely chopped fresh parsley**
- **¼ cup white wine vinegar**
- **2 tablespoons finely chopped onion**
- **3 cloves garlic, minced**
- **1 jalapeño pepper, finely chopped**
- **2 teaspoons dried oregano**

1. Prepare grill for direct cooking over medium heat.
2. Brush chicken with 4 teaspoons oil; season with salt and black pepper.
3. Grill chicken, covered, 6 to 8 minutes per side or until no longer pink in center (165°F).
4. Meanwhile, combine remaining ½ cup oil, parsley, vinegar, onion, garlic, jalapeño and oregano in small bowl; mix well. Season with salt and black pepper. Serve over chicken.

Tip

Chimichurri salsa can also be served with grilled steak or fish. Chimichurri will remain fresh tasting for 24 hours.

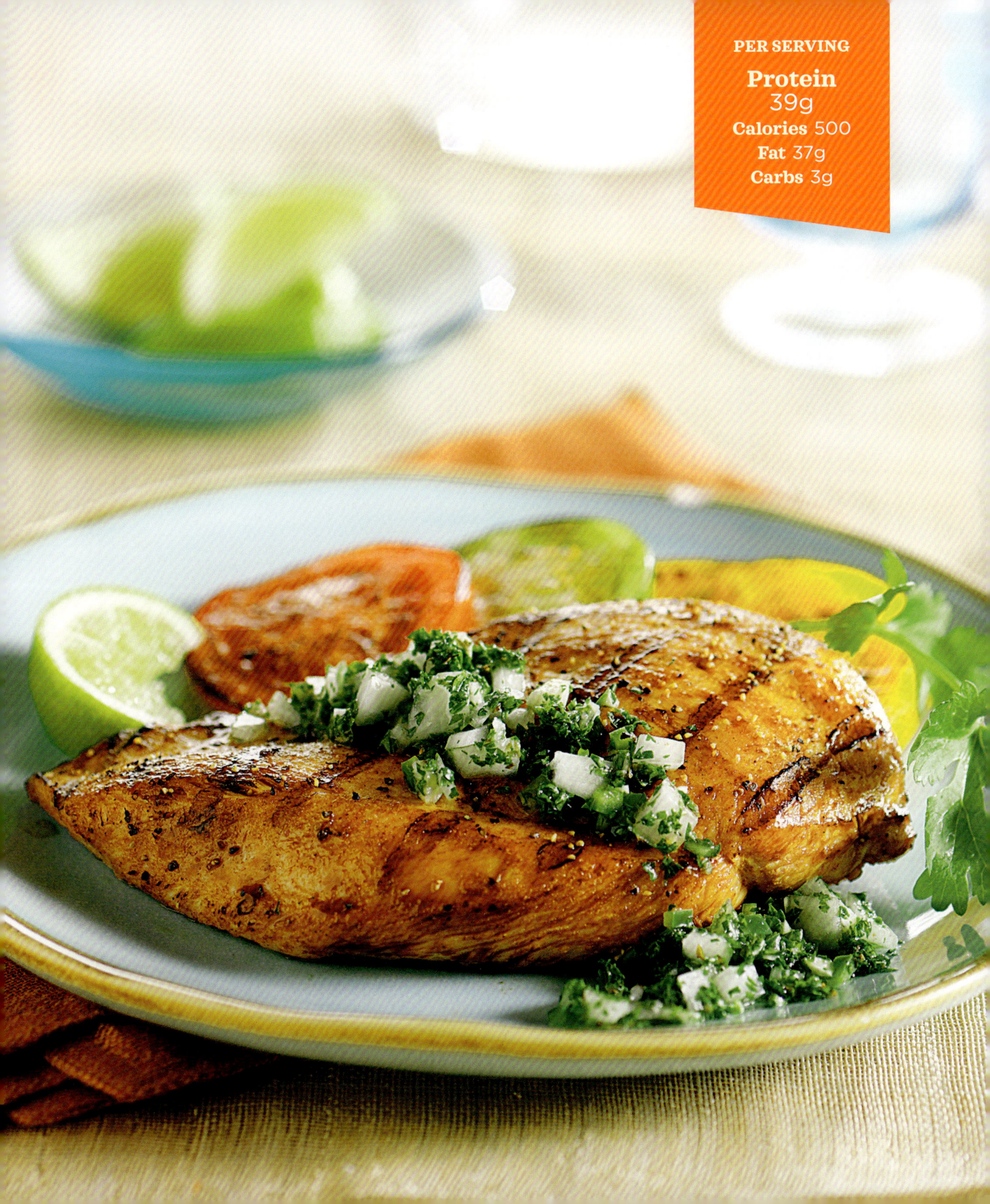
PER SERVING
Protein 39g
Calories 500
Fat 37g
Carbs 3g

Turkey Vegetable Skillet Lasagna

MAKES 6 SERVINGS

- **8 ounces hot Italian turkey sausage, casings removed**
- **8 ounces 93% lean ground turkey**
- **2 stalks celery, sliced**
- **⅓ cup chopped onion**
- **2 cups marinara sauce**
- **1⅓ cups water**
- **4 ounces uncooked bowtie (farfalle) pasta**
- **1 medium zucchini, halved lengthwise, then cut crosswise into ½-inch slices (2 cups)**
- **¾ cup chopped green or yellow bell pepper**
- **½ cup (2 ounces) shredded part-skim mozzarella cheese**
- **½ cup reduced-fat ricotta cheese**
- **2 tablespoons finely grated Parmesan cheese**

1. Heat large skillet over medium-high heat. Add sausage, ground turkey, celery and onion; cook and stir 6 to 8 minutes or until turkey is no longer pink.

2. Stir in marinara sauce and water; bring to a boil. Stir in pasta. Reduce heat to medium-low; cover and simmer 12 minutes, stirring occasionally.

3. Stir in zucchini and bell pepper; cover and cook 2 minutes. Uncover; cook 4 to 6 minutes or until vegetables are crisp-tender.

4. Sprinkle with mozzarella. Combine ricotta and Parmesan in small bowl; mix well. Drop by rounded teaspoonfuls over pasta mixture in skillet. Remove from heat; cover and let stand 10 minutes before serving.

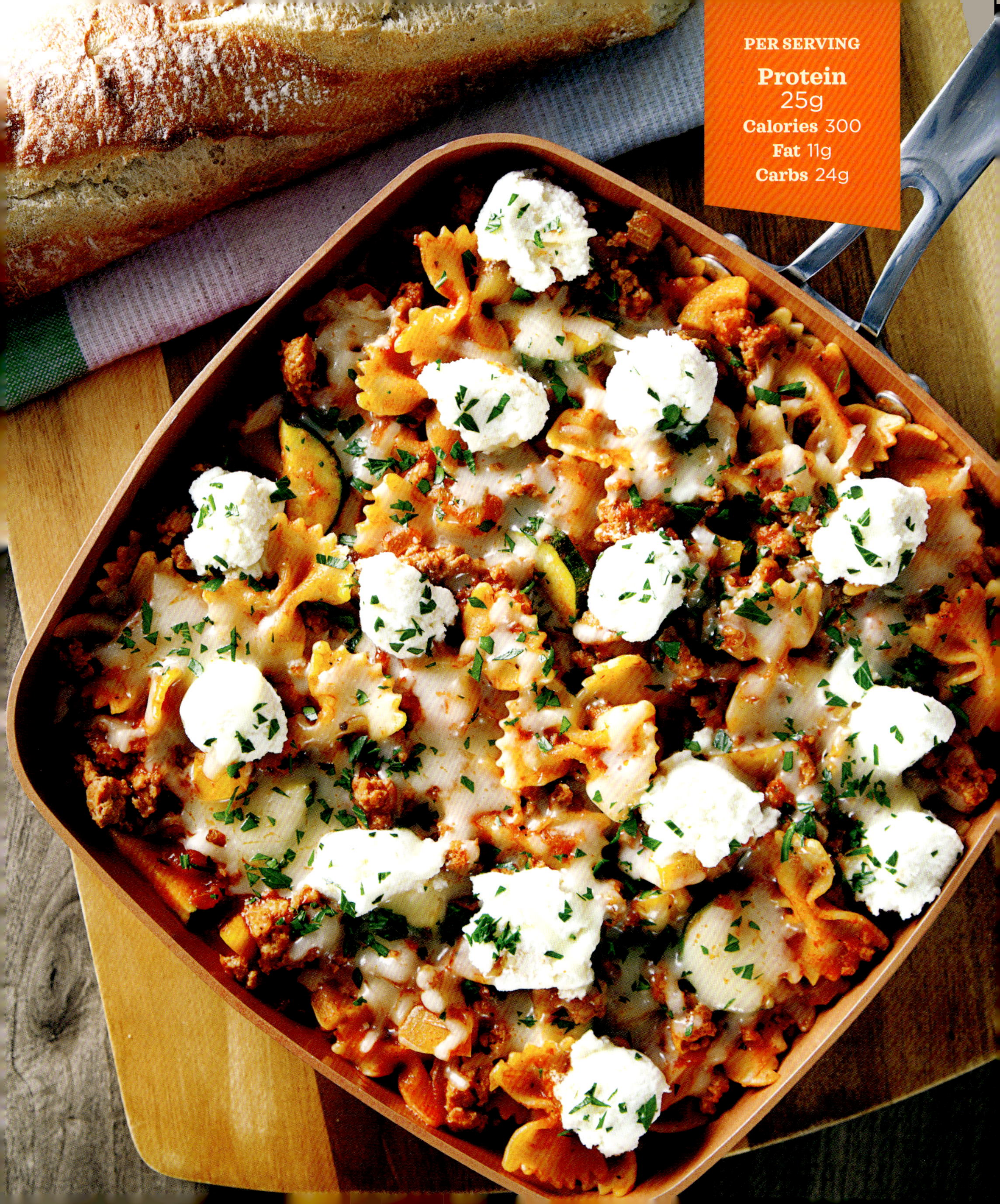
PER SERVING
Protein
25g
Calories 300
Fat 11g
Carbs 24g

Spiced Chicken Skewers with Yogurt-Tahini Sauce

MAKES 8 SERVINGS

- **1 cup plain nonfat or regular Greek yogurt**
- **¼ cup chopped fresh parsley, plus additional for garnish**
- **¼ cup tahini**
- **2 tablespoons lemon juice**
- **1 clove garlic**
- **¾ teaspoon salt, divided**
- **1 tablespoon vegetable oil**
- **2 teaspoons garam masala**
- **1 pound boneless skinless chicken breasts, cut into 1-inch pieces**

1. Prepare grill for direct cooking over medium-high heat. Spray grill grate with nonstick cooking spray.
2. Combine yogurt, ¼ cup parsley, tahini, lemon juice, garlic and ¼ teaspoon salt in food processor or blender; process until smooth.
3. Combine oil, garam masala and remaining ½ teaspoon salt in medium bowl; mix well. Add chicken; toss to coat. Thread chicken onto eight 6-inch wooden or metal skewers.*
4. Grill skewers 5 minutes per side or until chicken is cooked through. Serve with yogurt sauce; garnish with additional parsley.

**If using wooden skewers, soak in cold water 20 to 30 minutes to prevent burning.*

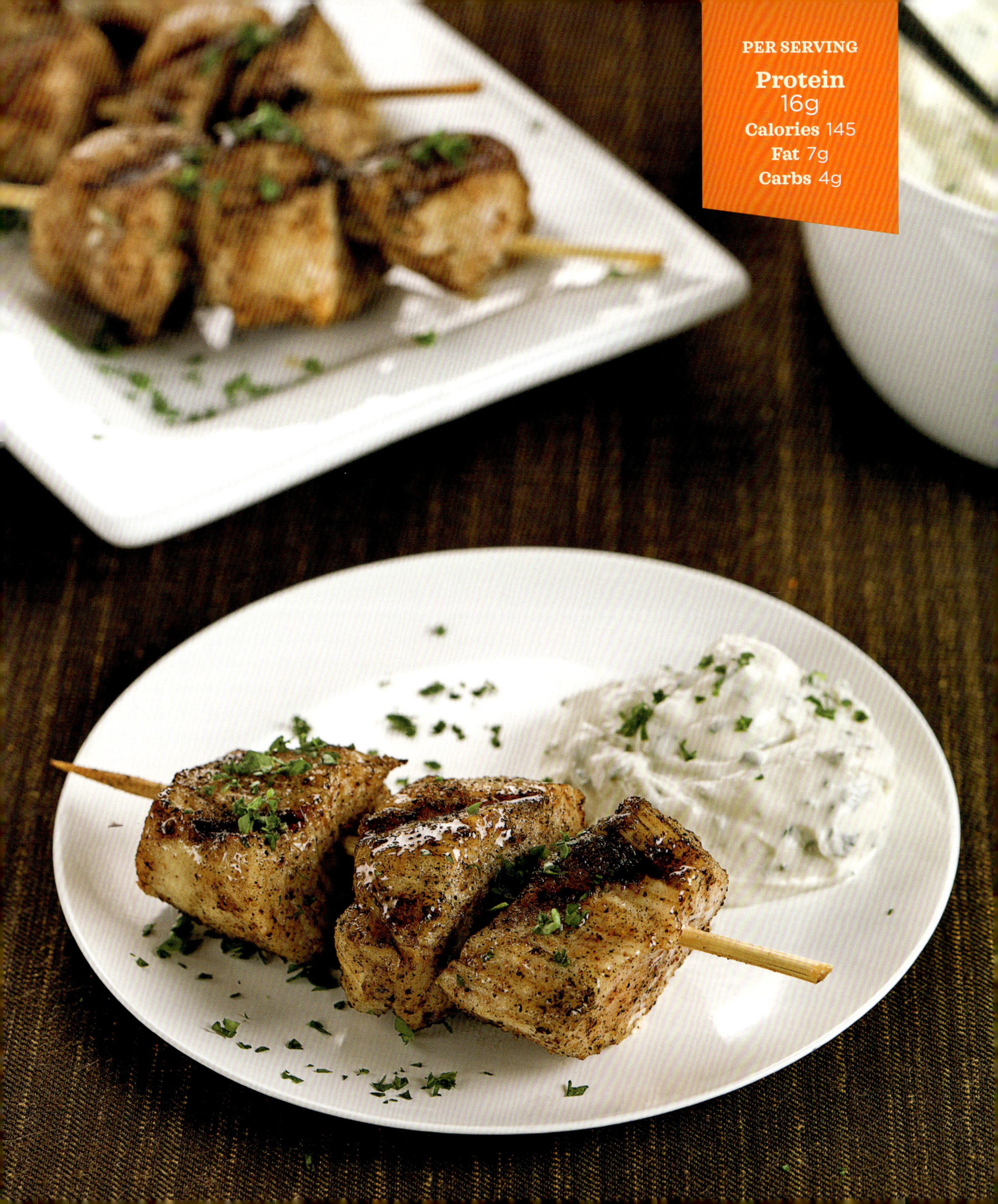
PER SERVING
Protein 16g
Calories 145
Fat 7g
Carbs 4g

PER SERVING
Protein
30g
Calories 250
Fat 9g
Carbs 17g

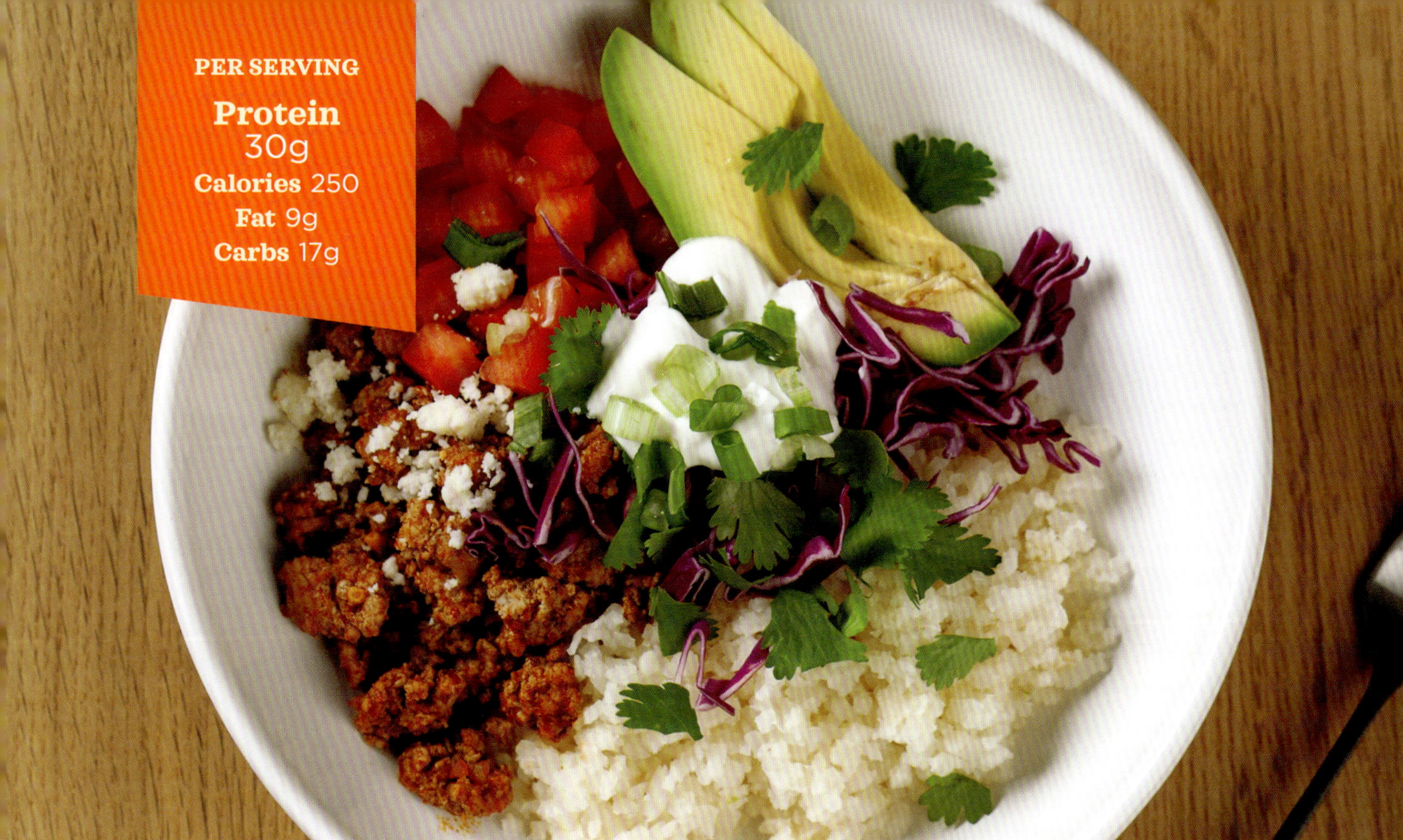

Turkey Taco Bowls

MAKES 4 SERVINGS

- 1 pound ground turkey
- 1 package (1 ounce) taco seasoning mix
- ¾ cup water
- 1 package (10 ounces) frozen cauliflower rice
- 2 cups shredded red cabbage
- 2 green onions, finely chopped
- 1 avocado, thinly sliced
- 2 plum tomatoes, diced
- Optional toppings: minced fresh cilantro, sour cream and crumbled cotija cheese

1. Cook turkey in large nonstick skillet over medium-high heat 6 to 8 minutes or until no longer pink, stirring to break up meat.
2. Stir in taco seasoning mix and water; bring to a boil. Reduce heat to medium-low; simmer 5 minutes, stirring occasionally.
3. Heat cauliflower rice according to package directions. Divide among four bowls; top with turkey, cabbage, green onions, avocado and tomatoes. Serve with desired toppings.

PER SERVING
Protein
32g
Calories 240
Fat 12g
Carbs 0g

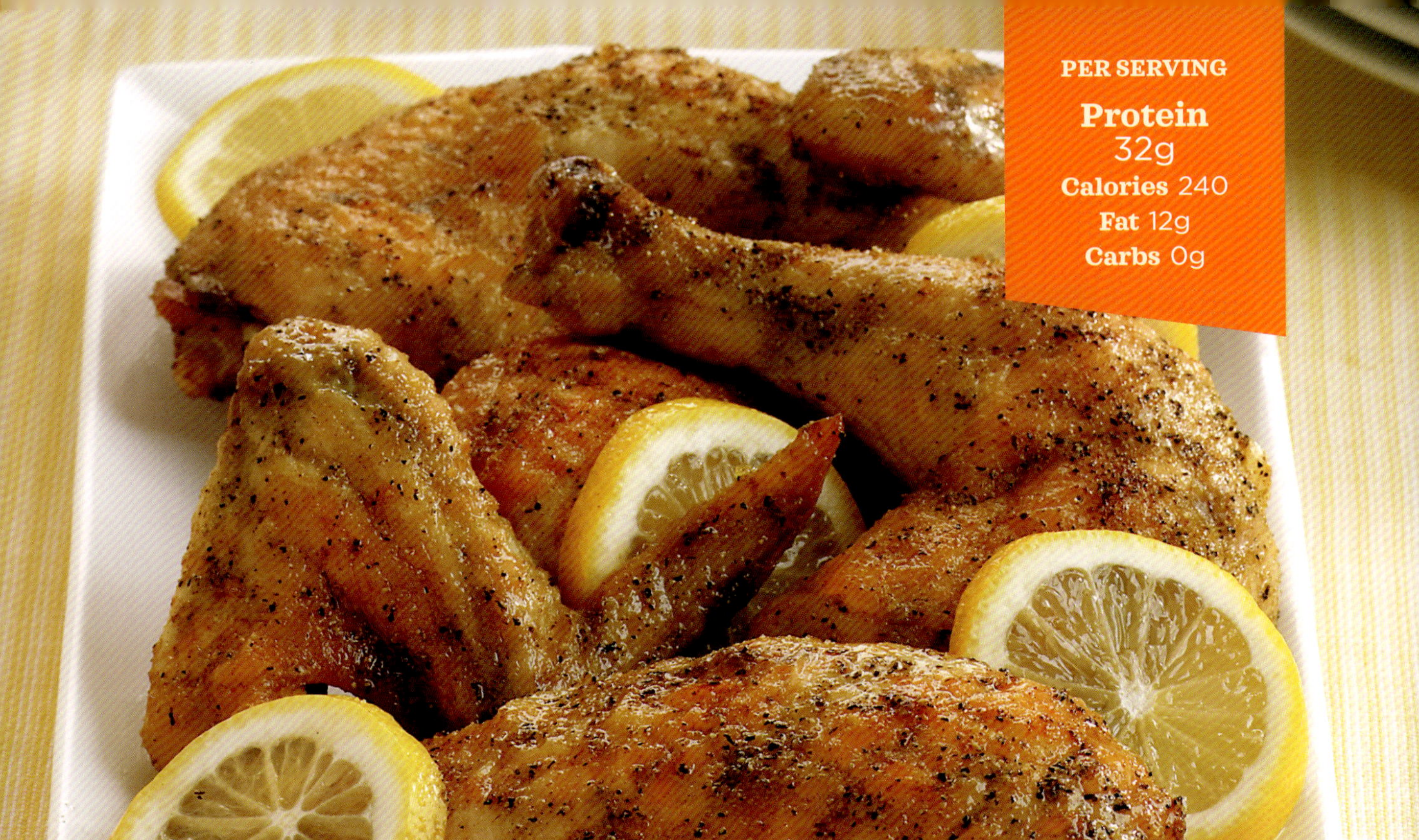

Lemony Greek Chicken

MAKES 4 SERVINGS

- 1 cut-up whole chicken (about 3 to 4 pounds)
- 1 tablespoon olive oil
- 2 teaspoons Greek seasoning
- 1 teaspoon salt
- 1 teaspoon black pepper
- Juice of 1 lemon

1. Preheat oven to 400°F.
2. Brush chicken with oil. Arrange in two large baking dishes, bone side down. Combine Greek seasoning, salt and pepper in small bowl; sprinkle half of mixture over chicken.
3. Bake 30 minutes. Turn chicken; sprinkle with remaining seasoning mixture and lemon juice. Bake 30 minutes or until chicken is cooked through (165°F).

Chicken Mirabella

MAKES 4 SERVINGS

- 4 boneless skinless chicken breasts (about 4 ounces each)
- ½ cup pitted prunes
- ½ cup assorted pitted olives (black, green or a combination)
- ¼ cup light white grape juice or dry white wine
- 2 tablespoons olive oil
- 1 tablespoon chopped fresh parsley, plus additional for garnish
- 1 tablespoon capers
- 1 tablespoon red wine vinegar
- 1 teaspoon dried oregano
- 1 clove garlic, minced
- 2 teaspoons packed brown sugar

1. Preheat oven to 350°F. Place chicken in 8-inch baking dish.

2. Combine prunes, olives, grape juice, oil, 1 tablespoon parsley, capers, vinegar, oregano and garlic in medium bowl; mix well. Pour over chicken; sprinkle with brown sugar.

3. Bake 25 to 30 minutes or until chicken is no longer pink in center (165°F), basting with sauce halfway through cooking. Garnish with additional parsley.

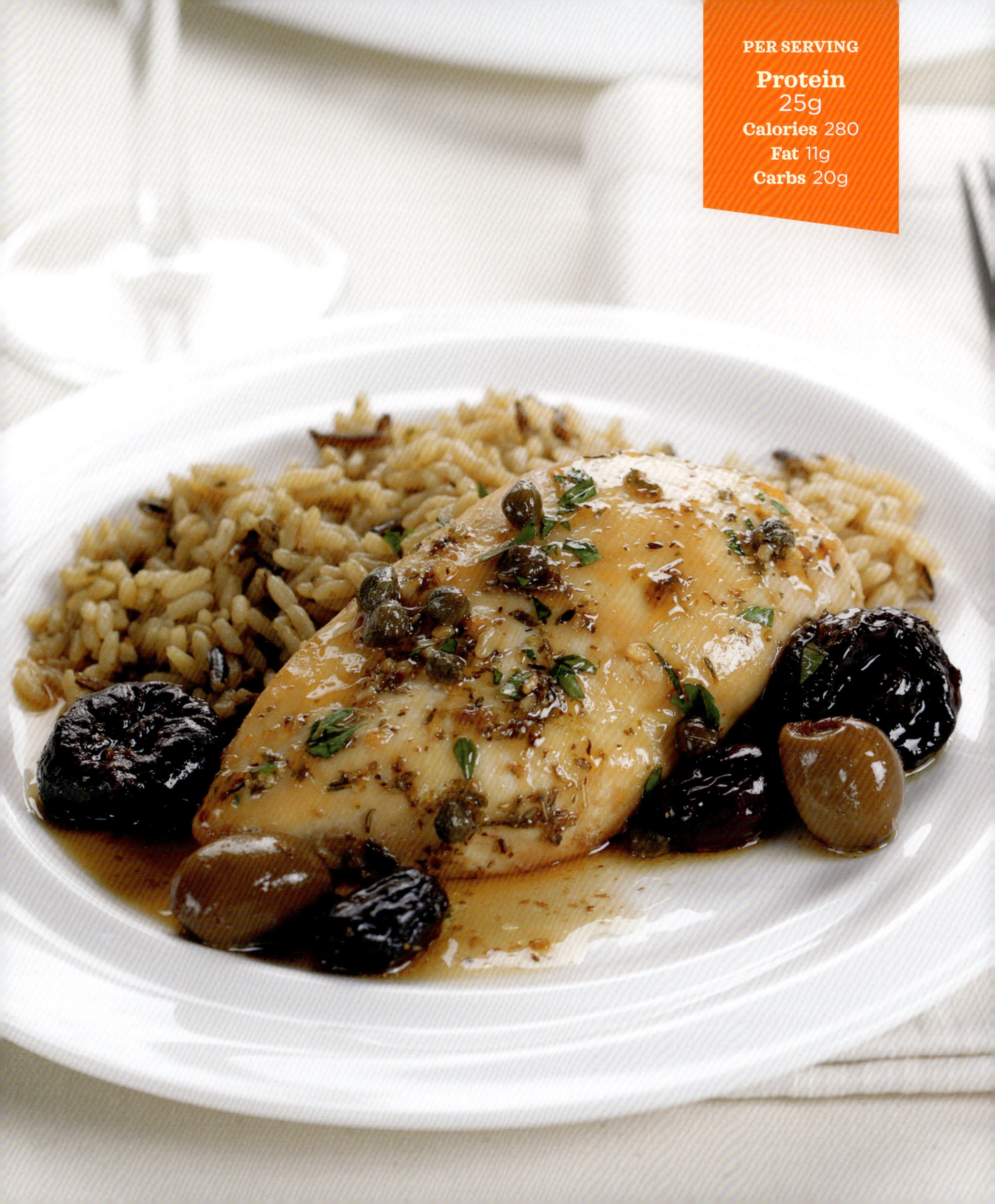
PER SERVING
Protein
25g
Calories 280
Fat 11g
Carbs 20g

Chicken with Curried Bulgur

MAKES 4 SERVINGS

- **1¼ cups water, divided**
- **½ teaspoon salt, divided**
- **½ cup uncooked bulgur wheat**
- **4 boneless skinless chicken breasts (about 4 ounces each)**
- **½ teaspoon ground cumin, divided**
- **¼ teaspoon black pepper**
- **¼ cup slivered almonds, toasted***
- **¼ cup raisins**
- **¼ cup chopped green onions, divided**
- **½ teaspoon grated fresh ginger**
- **½ teaspoon curry powder**

**To toast almonds, spread on small baking sheet; bake in preheated 350°F oven 5 to 7 minutes or until fragrant, stirring occasionally.*

1. Bring 1 cup water and ¼ teaspoon salt to a boil in small saucepan over high heat; stir in bulgur. Remove from heat; cover and let stand 10 minutes or until liquid is absorbed and bulgur is tender. Fluff with fork.

2. Meanwhile, sprinkle chicken with remaining ¼ teaspoon salt, ¼ teaspoon cumin and pepper. Spray large skillet with nonstick cooking spray; heat over medium-high heat. Add chicken; cook 4 to 5 minutes per side or until no longer pink in center (165°F). Remove to plate; tent with foil to keep warm.

3. Combine remaining ¼ cup water, ¼ teaspoon cumin, almonds, raisins, 2 tablespoons green onions, ginger and curry powder in same skillet; bring to a boil over medium-high heat, scraping up browned bits from bottom of skillet. Reduce heat to low; stir in bulgur until well blended.

4. Divide bulgur mixture among four plates. Top with chicken; sprinkle with remaining 2 tablespoons green onions.

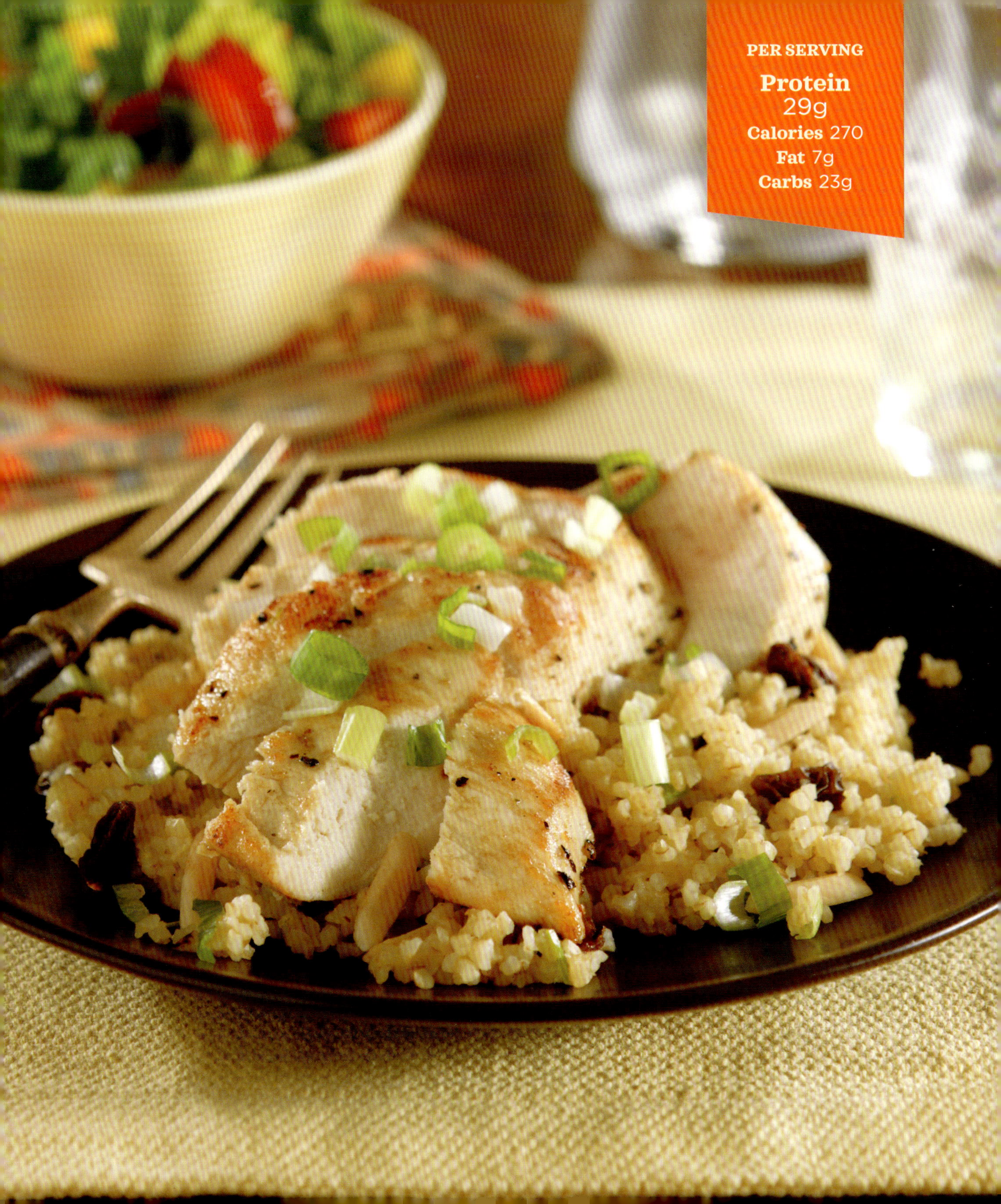
PER SERVING
Protein
29g
Calories 270
Fat 7g
Carbs 23g

PER SERVING
Protein
21g
Calories 180
Fat 9g
Carbs 1g

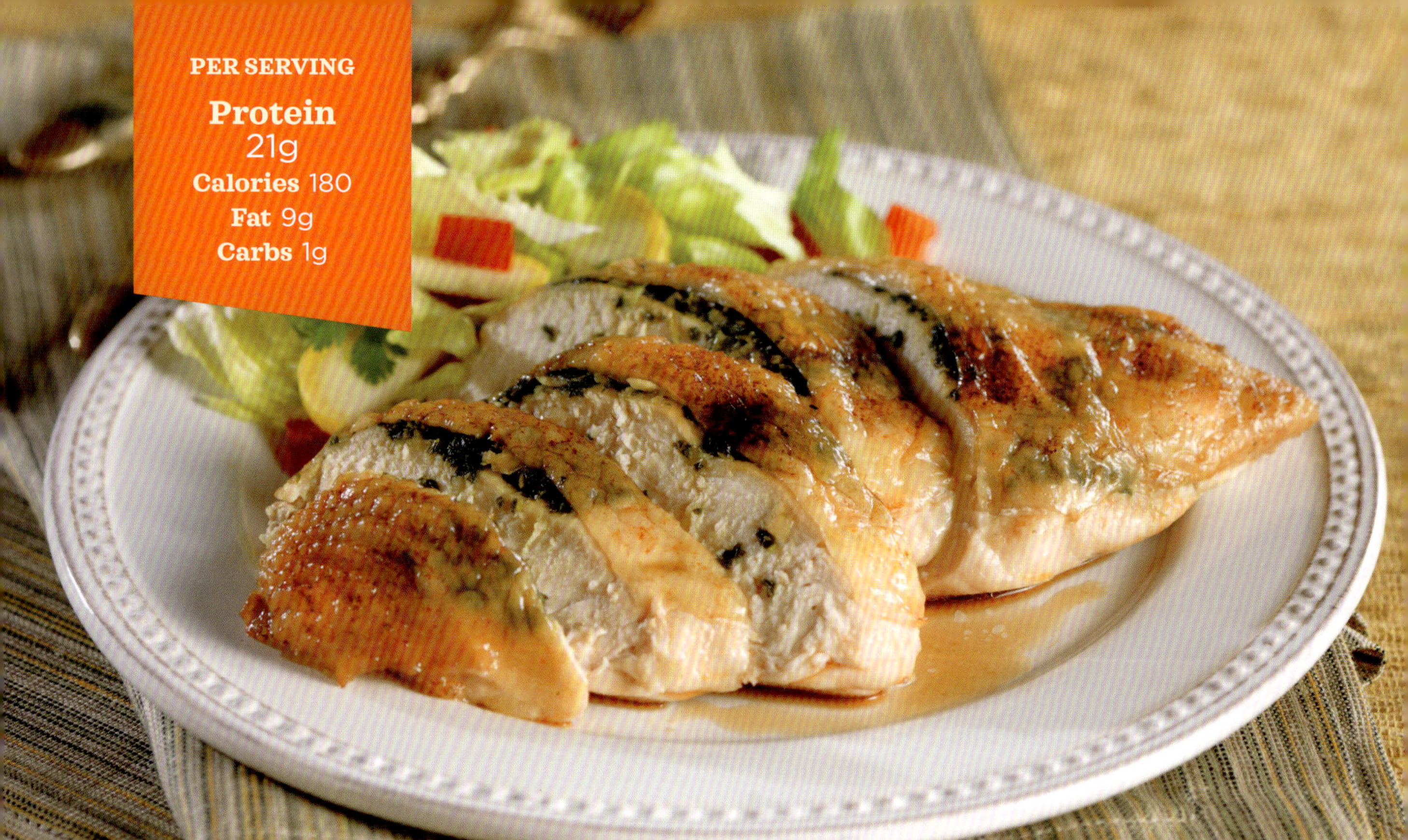

Cilantro-Stuffed Chicken Breasts

MAKES 4 SERVINGS

- 2 cloves garlic
- 1 cup packed fresh cilantro leaves
- 1 tablespoon plus 2 teaspoons soy sauce, divided
- 1 tablespoon peanut or vegetable oil
- 4 boneless chicken breasts (about 1¼ pounds)
- 1 tablespoon dark sesame oil

1. Preheat oven to 350°F. Line baking sheet or shallow baking pan with foil. Place wire rack over foil.

2. Mince garlic in small food processor or blender. Add cilantro; process until cilantro is finely chopped. Add 2 teaspoons soy sauce and peanut oil; process until paste forms. Spread about 1 tablespoon cilantro mixture evenly under skin of each chicken breast, being careful not to puncture skin.

3. Place chicken on wire rack. Combine remaining 1 tablespoon soy sauce and sesame oil in small bowl; brush half of mixture over chicken.

4. Bake 25 minutes. Brush with remaining soy sauce mixture; bake 10 minutes or until chicken is no longer pink in center (165°F).

PER SERVING
Protein
41g
Calories 350
Fat 3g
Carbs 40g

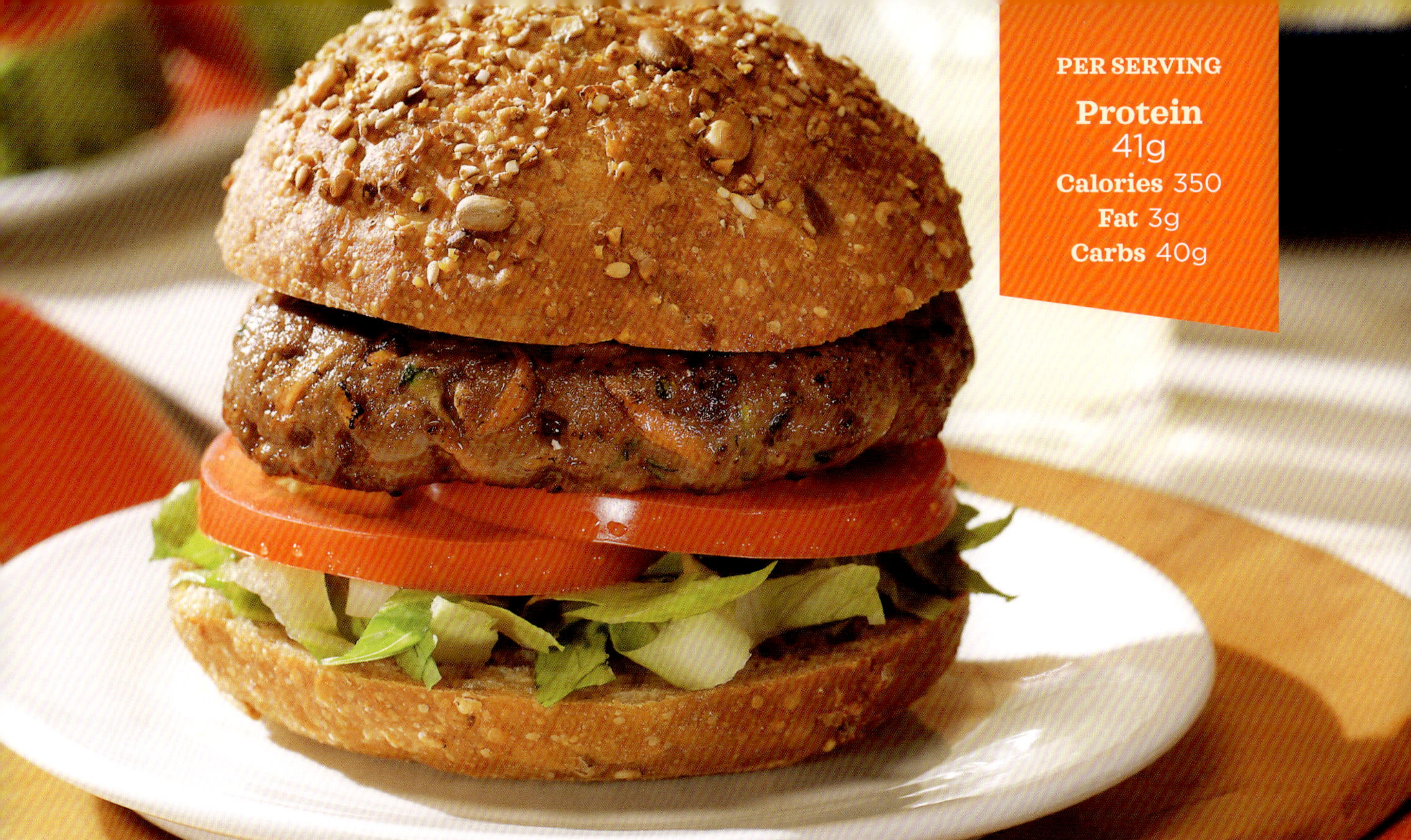

Veggie-Packed Turkey Burgers

MAKES 4 SERVINGS

- 1¼ pounds ground turkey
- ½ cup chopped onion
- ½ cup shredded zucchini
- ½ cup shredded carrots
- 1 teaspoon minced jalapeño pepper
- Salt and black pepper
- 4 whole wheat rolls or hamburger buns
- 1 cup shredded lettuce
- 8 tomato slices

1 Prepare grill for direct cooking over medium-heat. Spray grill grate with nonstick cooking spray.

2 Combine turkey, onion, zucchini, carrots and jalapeño in large bowl; mix gently. Season with salt and black pepper. Shape into four patties.

3 Grill patties, covered, 4 to 5 minutes per side or until cooked through (165°F).

4 Serve burgers on rolls with lettuce and tomato.

Cashew Chicken

MAKES 4 SERVINGS

- 10 ounces boneless skinless chicken breasts, cut into 1×½-inch pieces
- 1 tablespoon cornstarch
- 1 tablespoon dry white wine
- 1 tablespoon reduced-sodium soy sauce
- ½ teaspoon garlic powder
- 1 teaspoon vegetable oil
- 6 green onions, cut into 1-inch pieces
- 2 cups sliced mushrooms
- 1 red or green bell pepper, cut into strips
- 1 can (6 ounces) sliced water chestnuts, rinsed and drained
- 2 tablespoons hoisin sauce (optional)
- 2 cups hot cooked rice
- ¼ cup cashews, toasted*

**To toast cashews, cook in small skillet over medium heat 1 to 2 minutes or until lightly browned, stirring frequently.*

1 Place chicken in large resealable food storage bag. Whisk cornstarch, wine, soy sauce and garlic powder in small bowl until well blended and smooth. Pour over chicken; seal bag and turn to coat. Marinate in refrigerator 1 hour.

2 Drain chicken; discard marinade. Heat oil in wok or large nonstick skillet over medium-high heat. Add green onions; cook and stir 1 minute. Add chicken; cook and stir 2 minutes or until browned.

3 Add mushrooms, bell pepper and water chestnuts; cook and stir 3 minutes or until vegetables are crisp-tender and chicken is cooked through. Add hoisin sauce, if desired; cook and stir 1 minute or until heated through.

4 Serve chicken and vegetables over rice. Top with cashews.

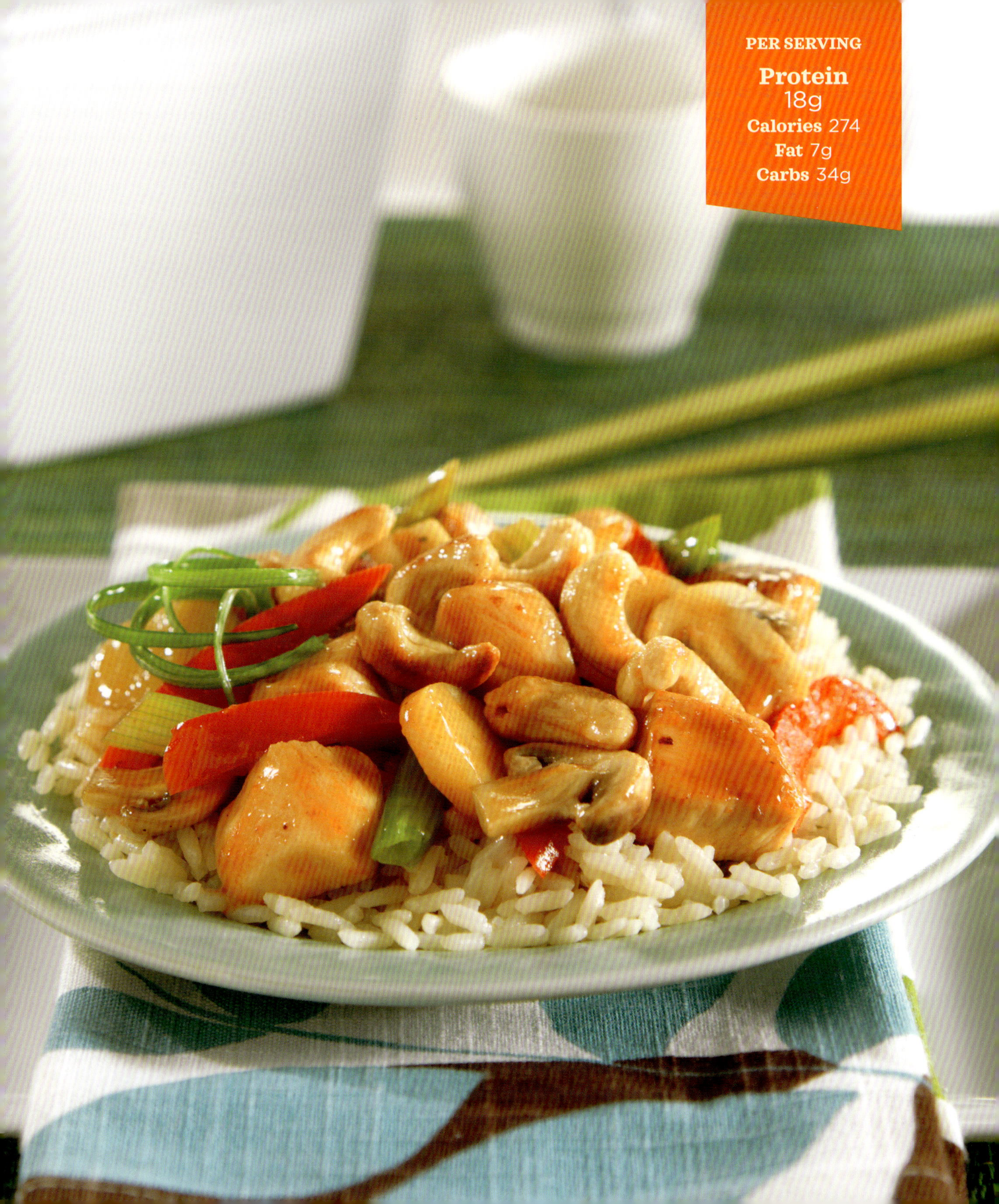

PER SERVING

Protein 18g

Calories 274

Fat 7g

Carbs 34g

PER SERVING
Protein
19g
Calories 370
Fat 8g
Carbs 49g

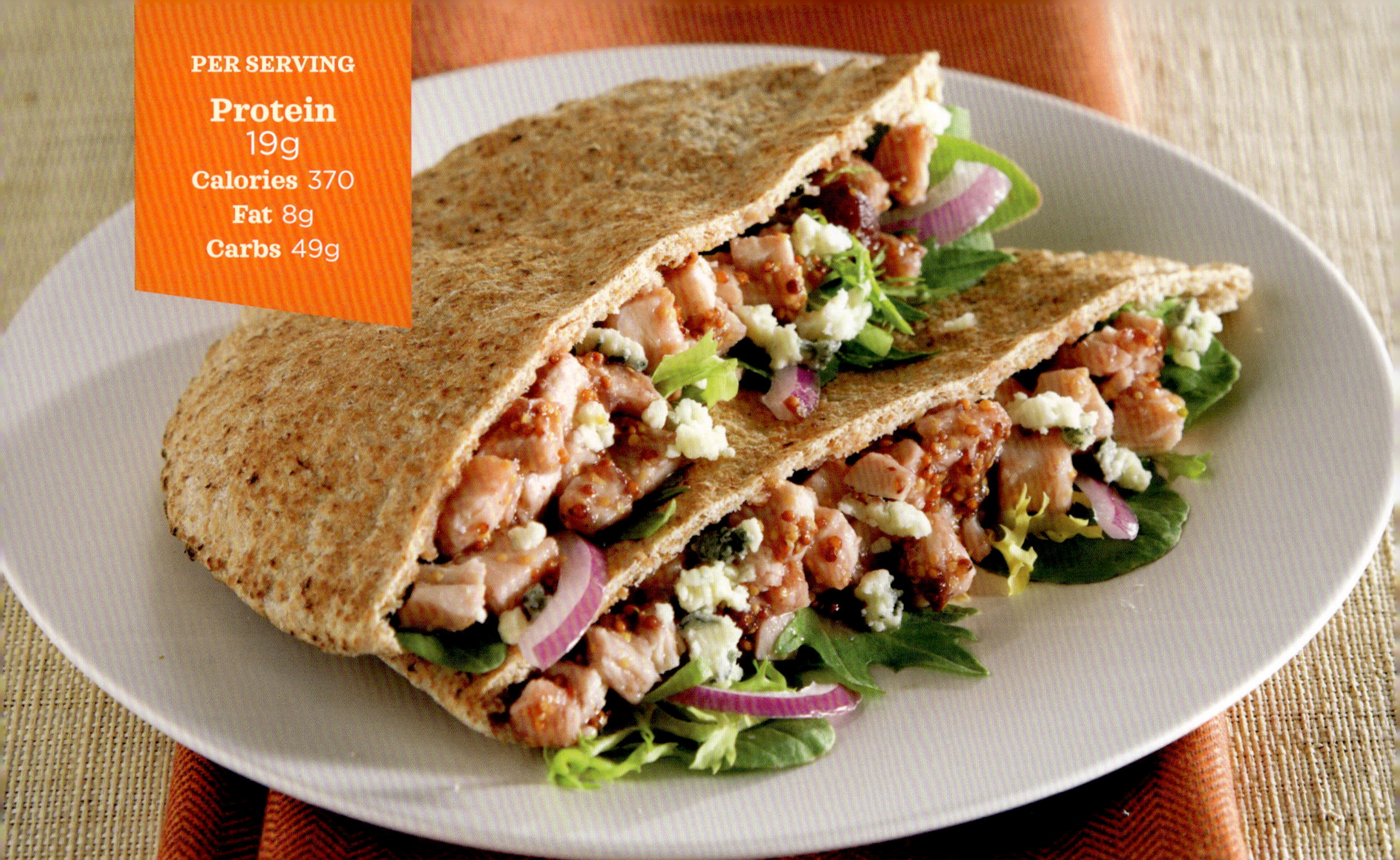

Stuffed Turkey Pitas with Cranberry Mustard and Blue Cheese

MAKES 4 SERVINGS

- ½ cup whole berry cranberry sauce
- 2 to 3 tablespoons coarse grain mustard
- 8 ounces chopped, cooked turkey breast (about 1 cup)
- 4 pita bread rounds, cut in half crosswise
- 4 cups packed mixed greens
- ½ cup thinly sliced red onion
- 2 ounces crumbled blue cheese

1 Whisk cranberry sauce and mustard in small bowl until well blended. Add turkey; stir to coat.

2 Fill each pita half with equal amounts of mixed greens, turkey, onion and cheese. Serve immediately.

PER SERVING
Protein
27g
Calories 260
Fat 2g
Carbs 34g

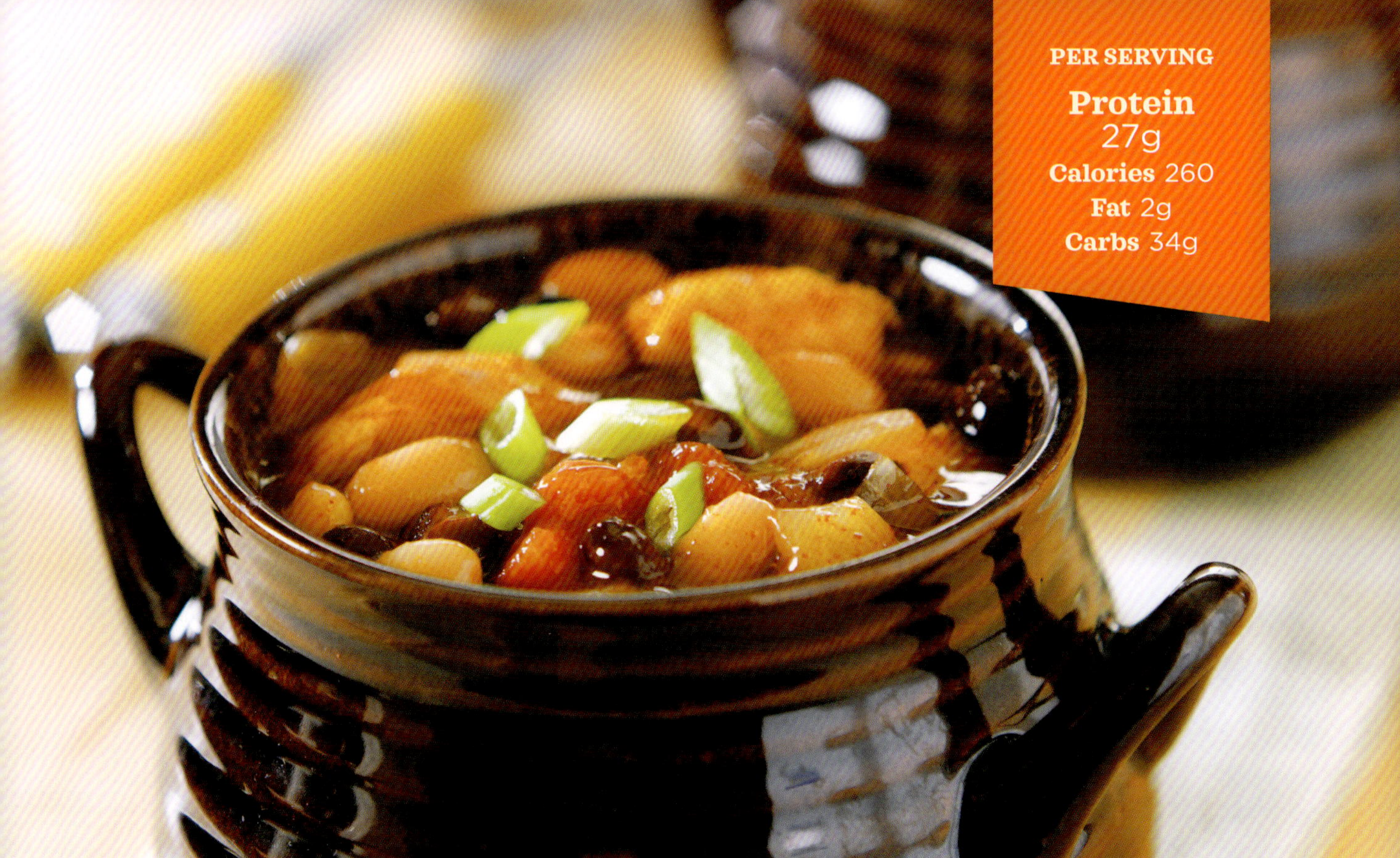

Black and White Chili

MAKES 6 SERVINGS

- 1 pound chicken tenders, cut into ¾-inch pieces
- 1 cup coarsely chopped onion
- 1 can (about 15 ounces) Great Northern beans, drained
- 1 can (about 15 ounces) black beans, drained
- 1 can (about 14 ounces) Mexican-style stewed tomatoes, undrained
- 2 tablespoons Texas-style chili seasoning mix

Slow Cooker Directions

1. Spray large skillet with nonstick cooking spray; heat over medium heat. Add chicken and onion; cook and stir 5 minutes or until chicken is browned.

2. Combine chicken mixture, beans, tomatoes with juice and chili seasoning in slow cooker; mix well.

3. Cover and cook on LOW 4 to 4½ hours.

Simple Roasted Chicken

MAKES 4 SERVINGS

- 1 whole chicken (about 4 pounds)
- 3 tablespoons butter, softened
- 1½ teaspoons salt
- 1 teaspoon onion powder
- 1 teaspoon dried thyme
- ½ teaspoon garlic powder
- ½ teaspoon paprika
- ½ teaspoon black pepper
- Fresh parsley sprigs and lemon wedges (optional)

1 Preheat oven to 425°F. Pat chicken dry; place in small baking pan or on baking sheet.

2 Combine butter, salt, onion powder, thyme, garlic powder, paprika and pepper in small microwavable bowl; mash with fork until well blended. Loosen skin on chicken breasts and thighs; spread about one third of butter mixture under skin.

3 Microwave remaining butter mixture until melted. Brush melted butter mixture all over outside of chicken and inside cavity. Tie drumsticks together with kitchen string and tuck wing tips under.

4 Roast 20 minutes. *Reduce oven temperature to 375°F.* Roast 45 to 55 minutes or until chicken is cooked through (165°F), basting once with pan juices during last 10 minutes of cooking. Remove chicken to cutting board; tent with foil and let stand 15 minutes before carving. Garnish with parsley and lemon wedges.

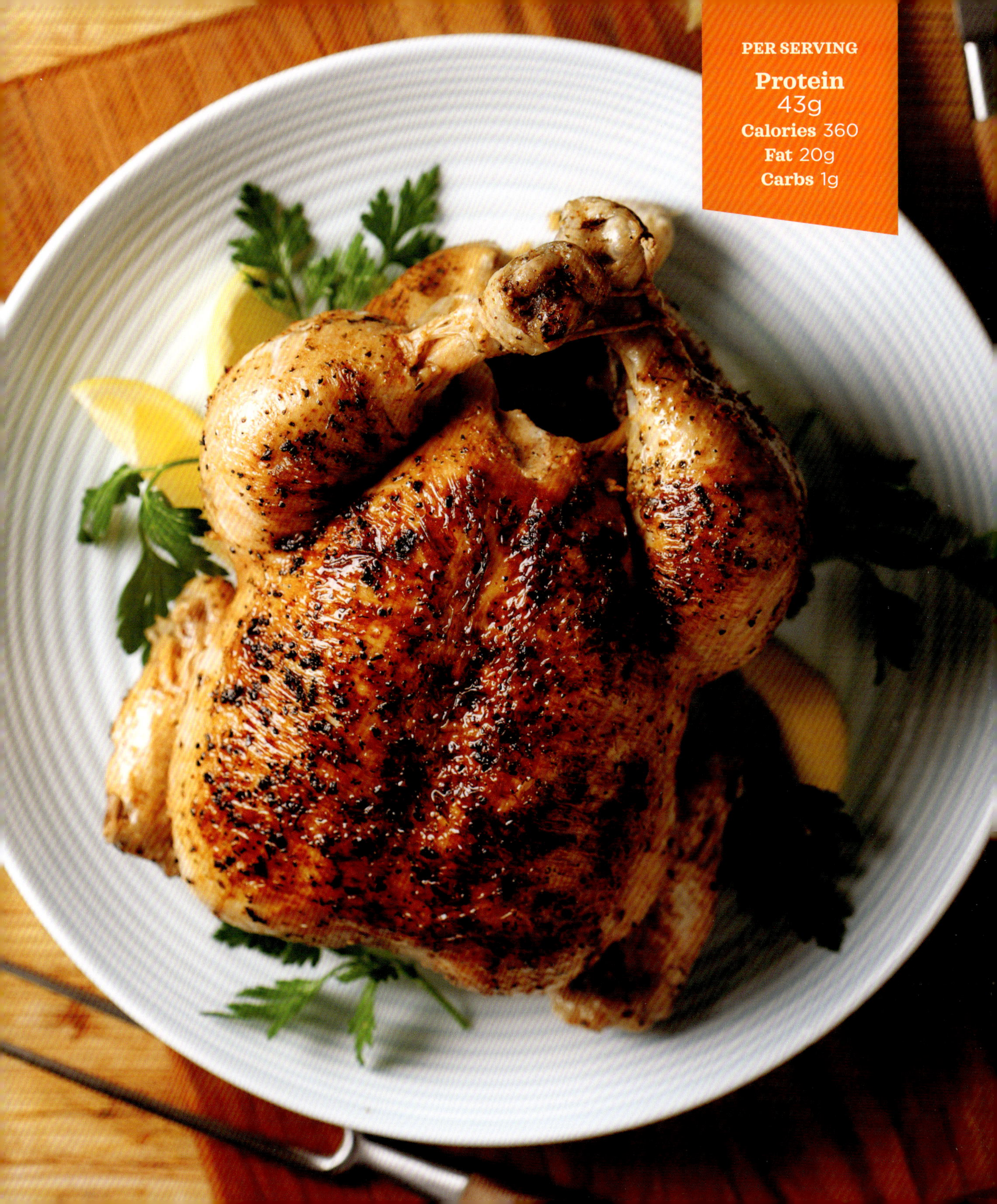
PER SERVING
Protein
43g
Calories 360
Fat 20g
Carbs 1g

Pesto Turkey Meatballs

MAKES 4 SERVINGS

- **1 pound ground turkey**
- **⅓ cup pesto sauce**
- **⅓ cup grated Parmesan cheese, plus additional for garnish**
- **¼ cup almond flour**
- **1 egg**
- **2 green onions, finely chopped**
- **½ teaspoon salt, divided**
- **2 tablespoons olive oil**
- **2 cloves garlic, minced**
- **⅛ teaspoon red pepper flakes**
- **1 can (28 ounces) whole tomatoes, undrained, crushed with hands or coarsely chopped**
- **1 tablespoon tomato paste**
- **Zucchini noodles (optional)**

1. Combine turkey, pesto, ⅓ cup cheese, almond flour, egg, green onions and ¼ teaspoon salt in medium bowl; mix gently. Shape mixture into 24 balls (about 1¼ inches). Refrigerate meatballs while preparing sauce.

2. Heat oil in large saucepan or Dutch oven over medium heat. Add garlic and red pepper flakes; cook and stir 2 minutes. Add tomatoes with juice, tomato paste and remaining ¼ teaspoon salt; cook 5 minutes or until sauce begins to simmer, stirring occasionally.

3. Remove about 1 cup sauce from saucepan. Arrange meatballs in single layer in saucepan; pour reserved sauce over meatballs. Reduce heat to medium-low; cover and cook 20 minutes.

4. Uncover; increase heat to medium-high. Cook about 10 minutes or until sauce thickens slightly and meatballs are cooked through (165°). Serve over zucchini noodles, if desired; garnish with additional cheese.

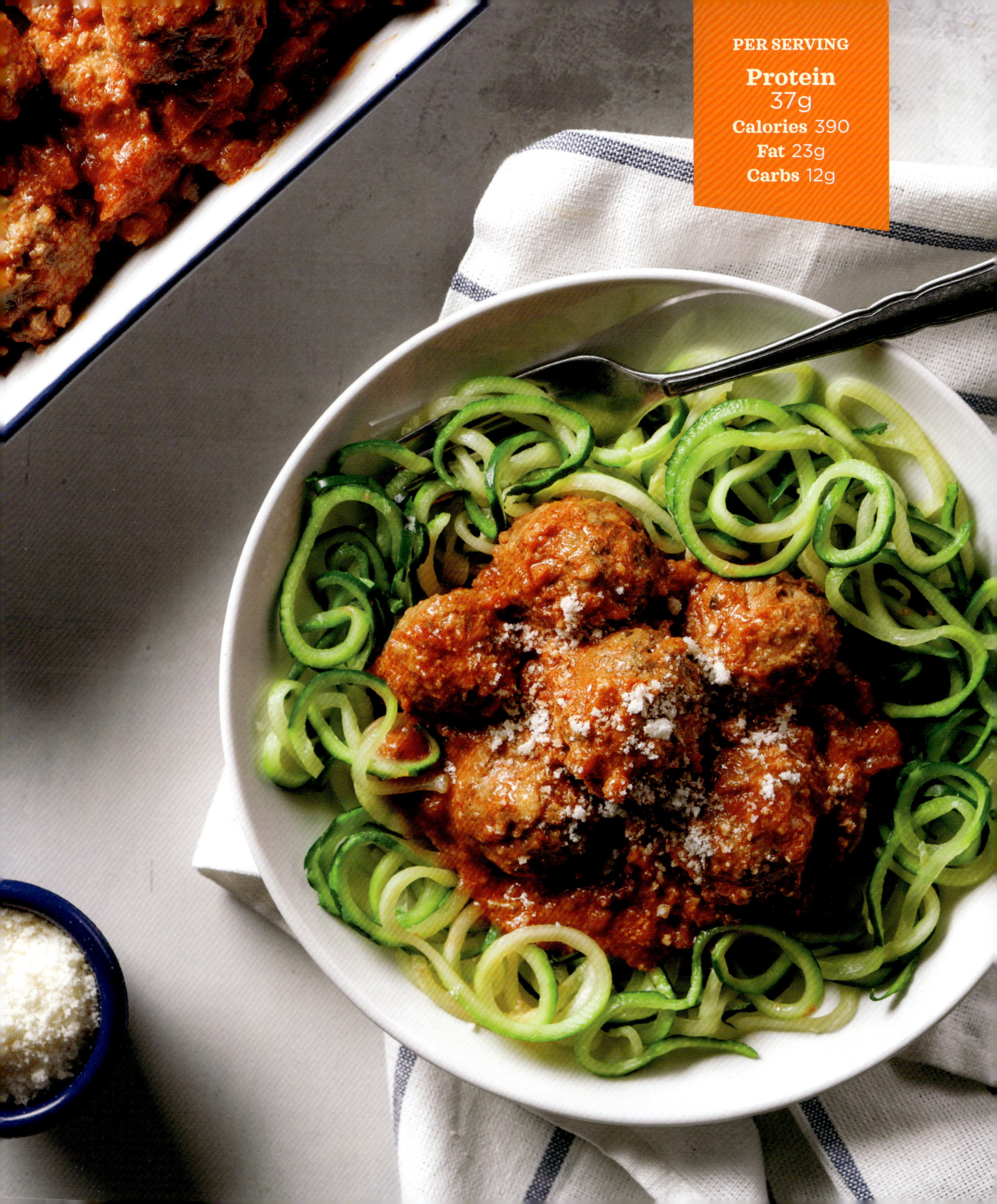
PER SERVING
Protein
37g
Calories 390
Fat 23g
Carbs 12g

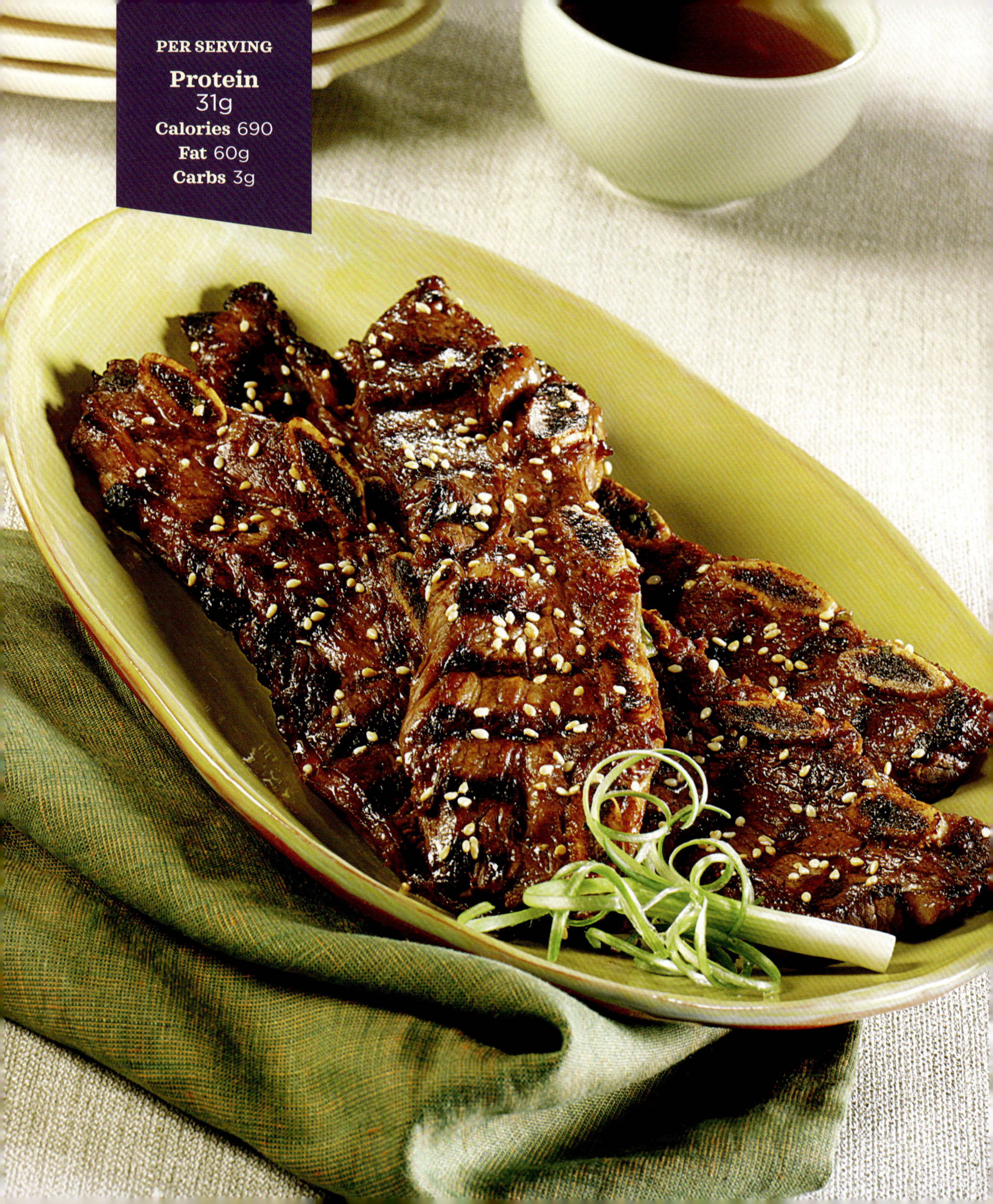
PER SERVING
Protein
31g
Calories 690
Fat 60g
Carbs 3g

MEAT

Korean Beef Short Ribs

MAKES 4 SERVINGS

- **2½ pounds beef chuck flanken-style short ribs (⅜ to ½ inch thick)***
- **¼ cup chopped green onions**
- **¼ cup water**
- **¼ cup soy sauce**
- **2 teaspoons grated fresh ginger**
- **2 teaspoons dark sesame oil**
- **2 cloves garlic, minced**
- **½ teaspoon black pepper**
- **1 tablespoon sesame seeds, toasted**

****Flanken-style ribs are available at Asian markets or they can be ordered from your butcher. They are cross-cut short ribs sawed through the bones.***

1 Place ribs in large resealable food storage bag. Combine green onions, water, soy sauce, ginger, oil, garlic and pepper in small bowl; mix well. Pour over ribs; seal bag and turn to coat. Marinate in refrigerator at least 4 hours or up to 8 hours, turning occasionally.

2 Prepare grill for direct cooking over medium-high heat. Remove ribs from marinade; reserve marinade.

3 Grill ribs, covered, 5 minutes. Brush lightly with reserved marinade; turn and brush again. Discard remaining marinade. Grill ribs, covered, 5 to 6 minutes for medium or to desired doneness. Sprinkle with sesame seeds.

Pork Tenderloin with Cabbage and Leeks

MAKES 4 SERVINGS

- **¼ cup olive oil, plus additional for pan**
- **1 teaspoon salt**
- **¾ teaspoon garlic powder**
- **½ teaspoon dried thyme**
- **½ teaspoon black pepper**
- **1 pork tenderloin (about 1¼ pounds)**
- **½ medium savoy cabbage, cored and cut into ¼-inch slices (about 6 cups)**
- **1 small leek, cut in half lengthwise and cut crosswise into ¼-inch slices**
- **1 to 2 teaspoons cider vinegar**

1 Preheat oven to 450°F. Brush baking sheet with oil.

2 Combine salt, garlic powder, thyme and pepper in small bowl; mix well. Stir in ¼ cup oil until well blended. Brush pork with about 1 tablespoon oil mixture, turning to coat all sides.

3 Combine cabbage and leek in large bowl. Drizzle with remaining oil mixture; toss to coat. Spread on prepared baking sheet; top with pork.

4 Bake 25 minutes or until pork is 145°F, stirring cabbage mixture halfway through cooking. Remove pork to cutting board; tent with foil to keep warm. Let stand 10 minutes before slicing. Add vinegar to cabbage mixture; stir to blend.

Tip

If you can't find savoy cabbage, you can substitute regular green cabbage but it may take slightly longer to cook. If the cabbage is not crisp-tender when the pork is done, return the vegetables to the oven for 10 minutes or until crisp-tender.

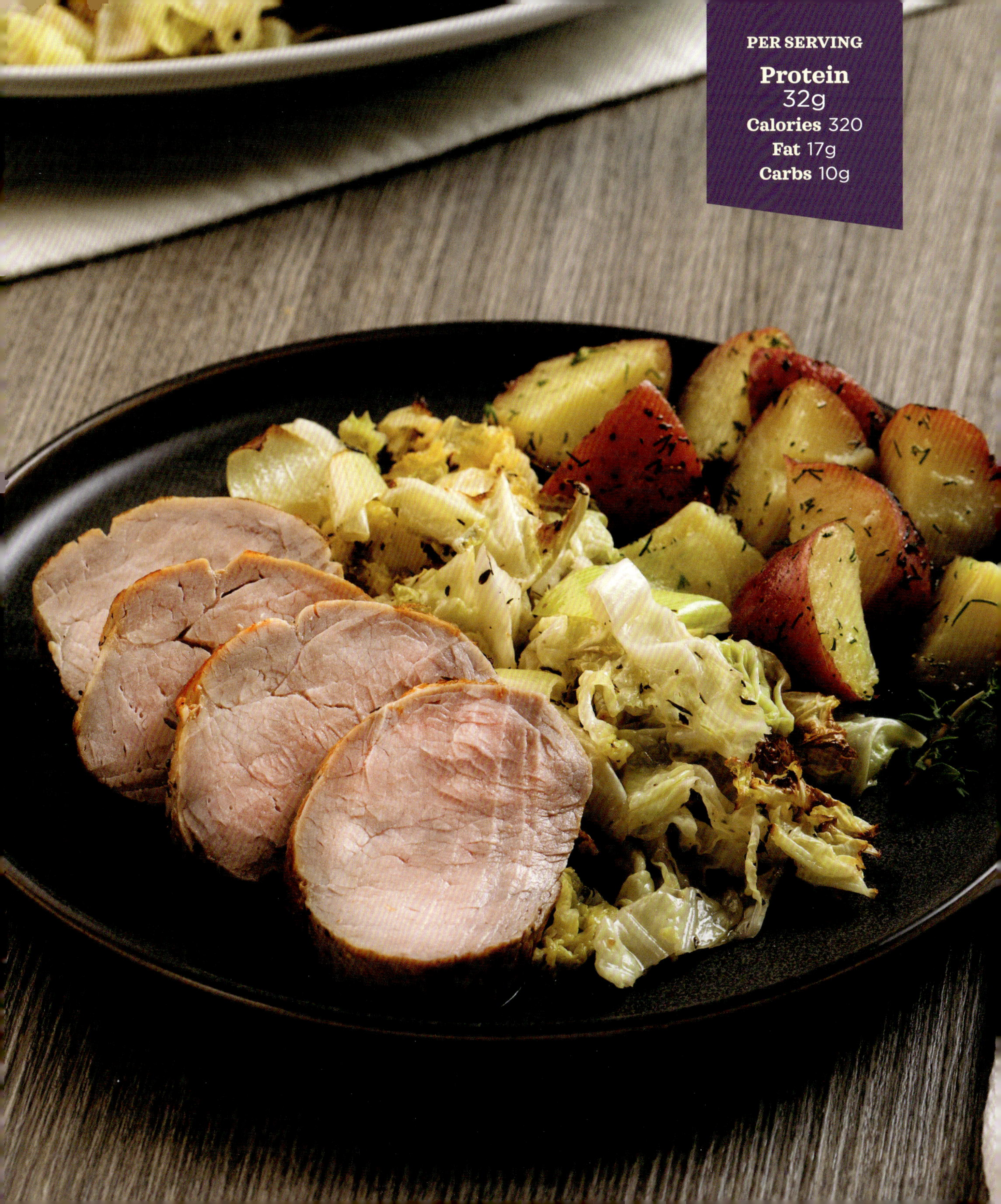
PER SERVING
Protein
32g
Calories 320
Fat 17g
Carbs 10g

Red Wine Oregano Beef Kabobs

MAKES 4 SERVINGS

- **12 ounces boneless beef top sirloin steak, cut into 16 (1-inch) pieces**
- **16 whole mushrooms (about 8 ounces total)**
- **1 medium red onion, cut in eight wedges and layers separated**
- **¼ cup dry red wine**
- **¼ cup finely chopped fresh parsley**
- **2 tablespoons Worcestershire sauce**
- **1 tablespoon reduced-sodium soy sauce**
- **3 cloves garlic, minced**
- **1 teaspoon dried oregano**
- **½ teaspoon salt (optional)**
- **½ teaspoon black pepper**

1. Combine steak, mushrooms and onion in large resealable food storage bag. Combine wine, parsley, Worcestershire sauce, soy sauce, garlic, oregano, salt, if desired, and pepper in small bowl; mix well. Pour over steak and vegetables; seal bag and turn to coat. Marinate in refrigerator 1 hour, turning frequently.

2. Soak four 12-inch or eight 6-inch bamboo skewers in cold water 20 to 30 minutes to prevent burning.

3. Preheat broiler. Spray broiler rack with nonstick cooking spray.

4. Alternately thread steak, mushrooms and onion onto skewers. Place skewers on prepared broiler rack; brush with marinade.

5. Broil 4 to 6 inches from heat source 8 to 10 minutes, turning occasionally.

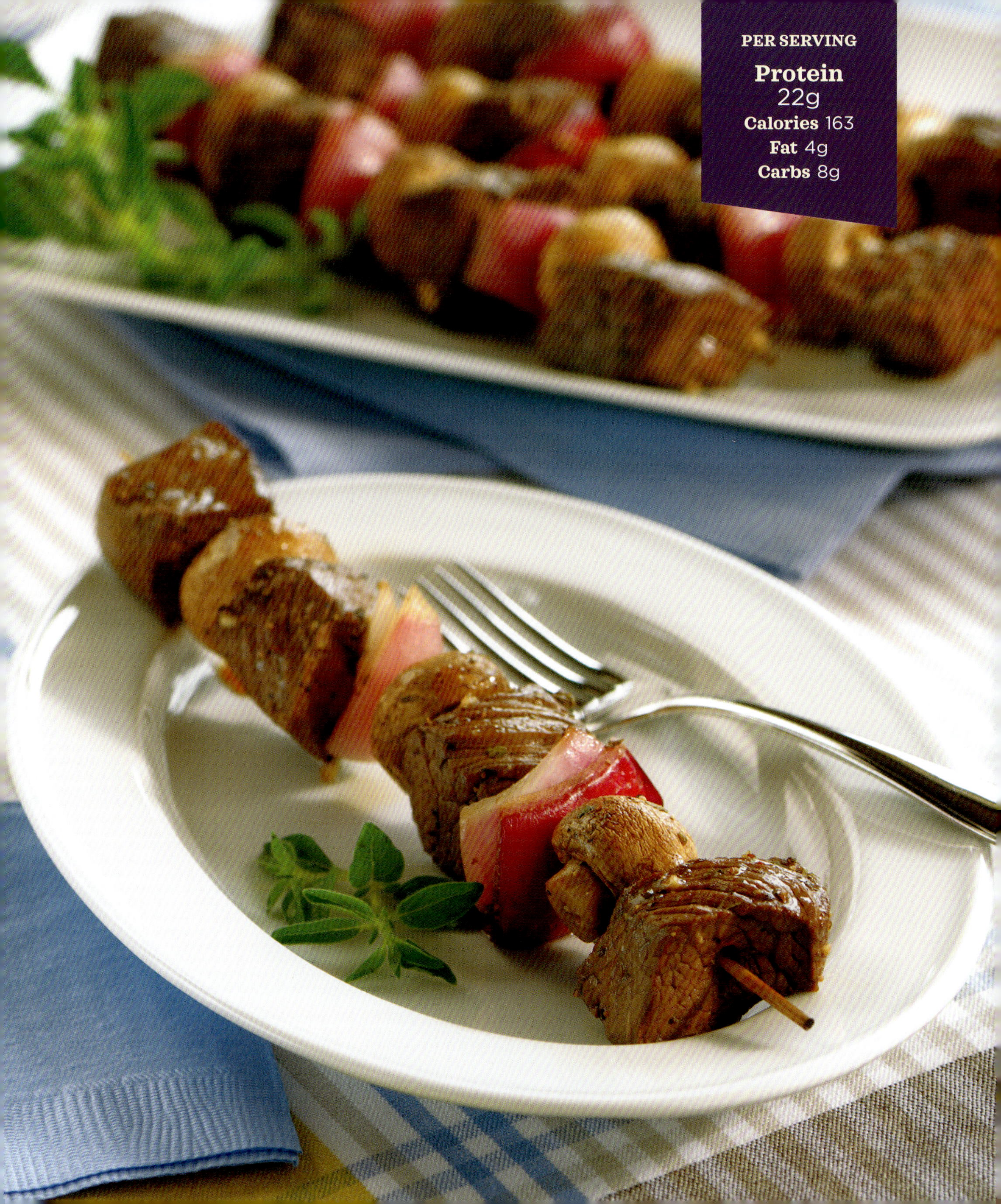
PER SERVING
Protein
22g
Calories 163
Fat 4g
Carbs 8g

Herbed Lamb Chops

MAKES 4 TO 6 SERVINGS

- 8 lamb loin chops, 1 inch thick (about 2 pounds)
- ⅓ cup vegetable oil
- ⅓ cup red wine vinegar
- 2 tablespoons soy sauce
- 1 tablespoon lemon juice
- 3 cloves garlic, minced
- 1 teaspoon salt
- 1 teaspoon chopped fresh oregano *or* ¼ teaspoon dried oregano
- 1 teaspoon dried rosemary
- 1 teaspoon ground mustard
- ½ teaspoon white pepper

1 Place lamb in large resealable food storage bag. Whisk oil, vinegar, soy sauce, lemon juice, garlic, salt, oregano, rosemary, mustard and pepper in medium bowl until well blended.

2 Reserve ½ cup marinade in small bowl. Pour remaining marinade over lamb; seal bag and turn to coat. Marinate in refrigerator at least 1 hour.

3 Prepare grill for direct cooking over medium-high heat. Remove lamb from marinade; discard marinade.

4 Grill lamb about 4 minutes per side or to desired doneness, turning once and basting often with reserved ½ cup marinade. (Do not baste during last 5 minutes of cooking.) Discard any remaining marinade.

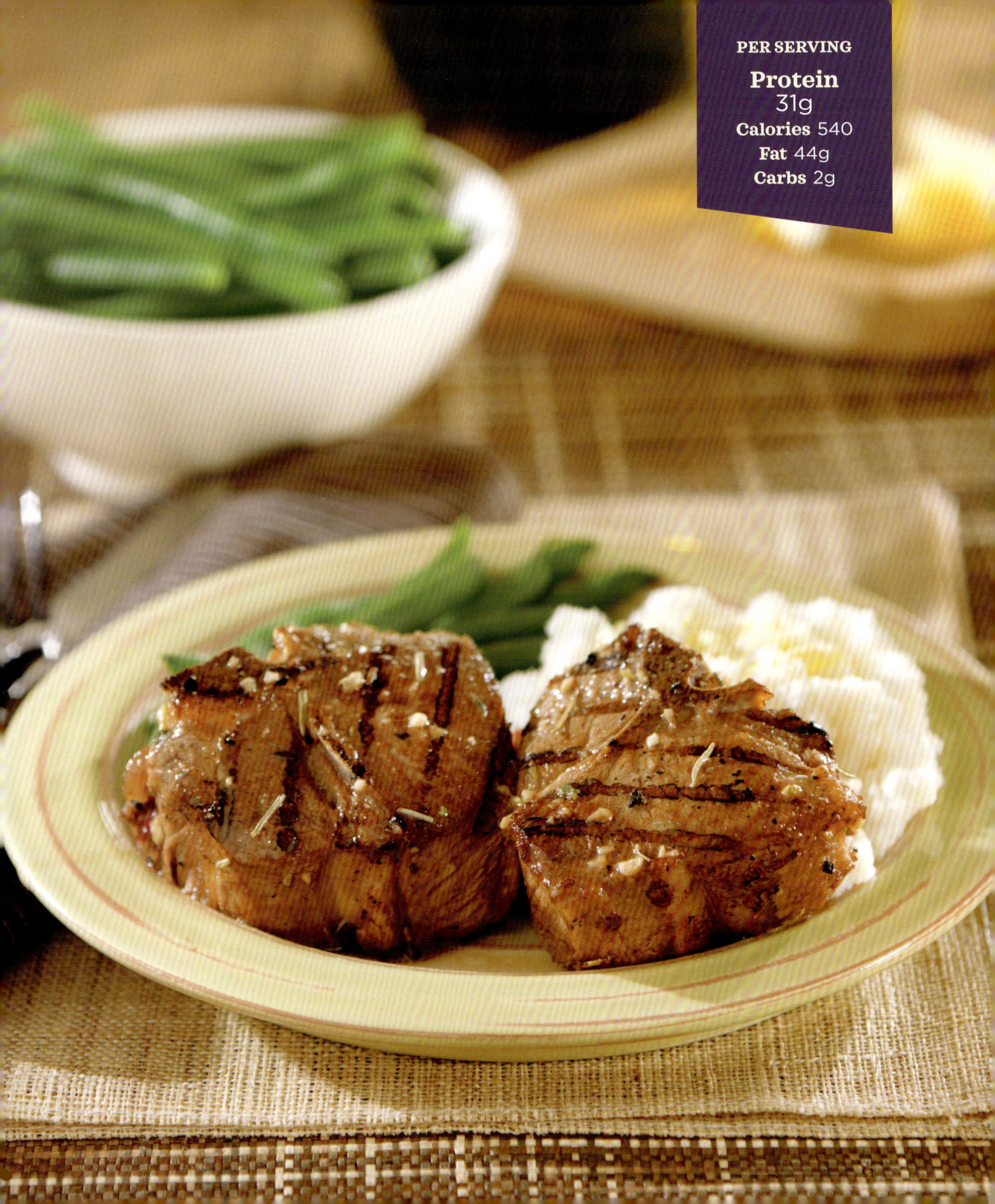
PER SERVING
Protein
31g
Calories 540
Fat 44g
Carbs 2g

Steak Fajitas

MAKES 4 SERVINGS

- 1 pound flank steak, skirt steak or top sirloin
- ¼ cup lime juice
- ¼ cup soy sauce
- 4 tablespoons vegetable oil, divided
- 2 tablespoons honey
- 2 tablespoons Worcestershire sauce
- 2 cloves garlic, minced
- ½ teaspoon ground red pepper
- 1 medium yellow onion, halved and cut into ¼-inch slices
- 1 green bell pepper, cut into ¼-inch strips
- 1 red bell pepper, cut into ¼-inch strips
- Flour tortillas and lime wedges (optional)
- Optional toppings: pico de gallo, guacamole and sour cream

1. Place steak in large resealable food storage bag. Combine lime juice, soy sauce, 2 tablespoons oil, honey, Worcestershire sauce, garlic and ground red pepper in medium bowl; mix well.

2. Remove ¼ cup marinade to large bowl. Pour remaining marinade over steak; seal bag and turn to coat. Marinate in refrigerator at least 2 hours or overnight. Add onion and bell peppers to bowl with ¼ cup marinade; toss to coat. Cover and refrigerate until ready to use.

3. Remove steak from marinade; discard marinade and pat steak dry with paper towel. Heat 1 tablespoon oil in large skillet (preferably cast iron) over medium-high heat. Cook steak about 4 minutes per side for medium rare or to desired doneness. Remove to cutting board; tent with foil and let rest 10 minutes.

4. Meanwhile, heat remaining 1 tablespoon oil in same skillet over medium-high heat. Add vegetable mixture; cook about 8 minutes or until vegetables are crisp-tender and beginning to brown in spots, stirring occasionally. (Cook in two batches if necessary; do not pile vegetables in skillet.)

5. Cut steak into thin slices across the grain. Serve with vegetables, tortillas, lime wedges and desired toppings.

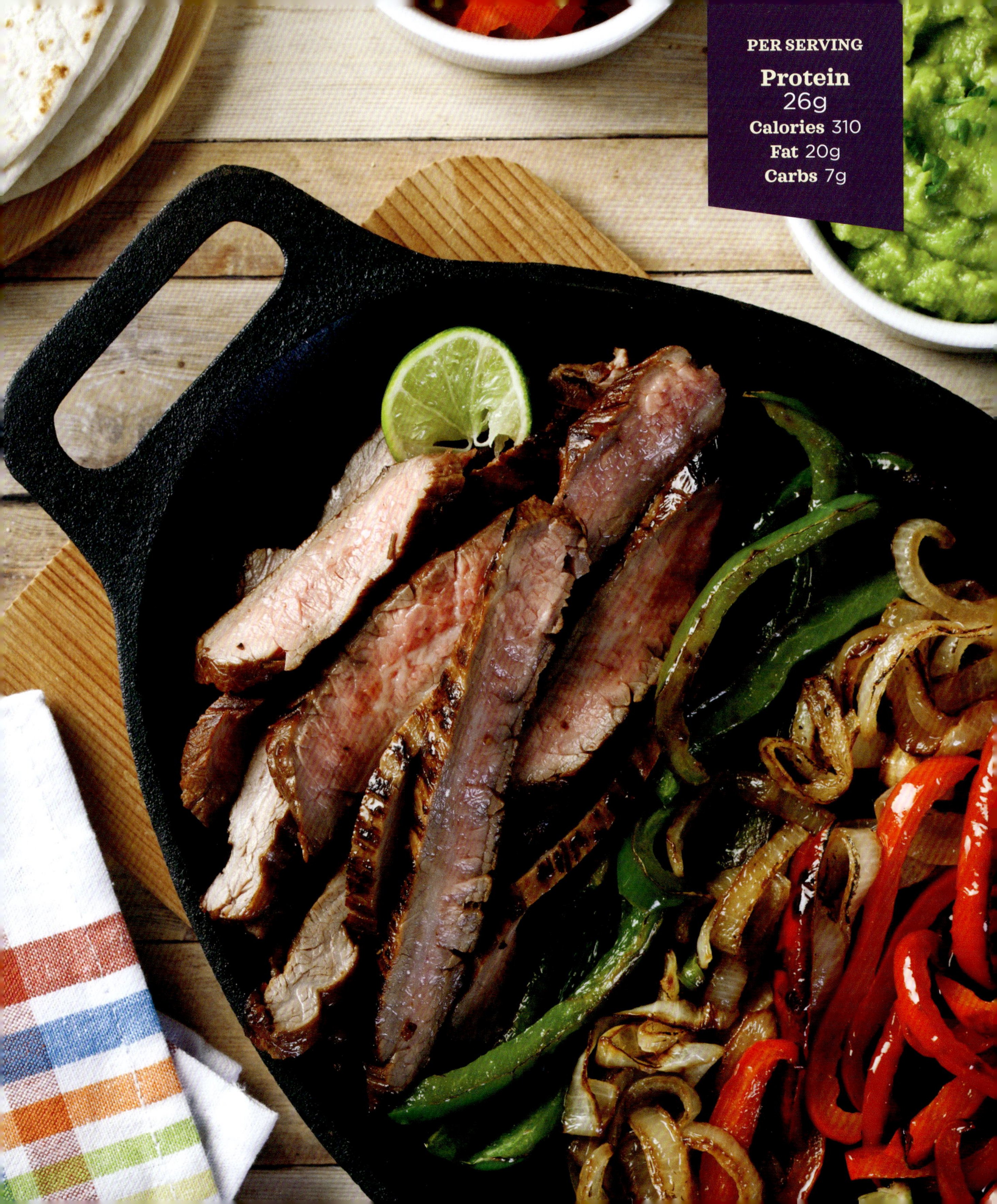
PER SERVING
Protein
26g
Calories 310
Fat 20g
Carbs 7g

Zesty Skillet Pork Chops

MAKES 4 SERVINGS

- **1 teaspoon chili powder**
- **½ teaspoon salt, divided**
- **4 lean boneless pork chops (about 5 ounces each)**
- **2 cups diced tomatoes**
- **1 cup chopped green, red or yellow bell pepper**
- **¾ cup thinly sliced celery**
- **½ cup chopped onion**
- **1 tablespoon hot pepper sauce**
- **1 teaspoon dried thyme**
- **2 tablespoons finely chopped fresh parsley**

1. Combine chili powder and ¼ teaspoon salt; sprinkle over one side of pork chops.
2. Combine tomatoes, bell pepper, celery, onion, hot pepper sauce and thyme in medium bowl; mix well.
3. Lightly spray large nonstick skillet with nonstick cooking spray; heat over medium-high heat. Add pork, seasoned side down; cook 1 minute. Turn pork; top with tomato mixture and bring to a boil. Reduce heat to low; cover and cook 25 minutes or until pork is tender and tomato mixture has thickened.
4. Remove pork to serving plates. Bring tomato mixture to a boil over high heat; cook 2 minutes or until most of liquid has evaporated.
5. Remove from heat; stir in parsley and remaining ¼ teaspoon salt. Spoon sauce over pork.

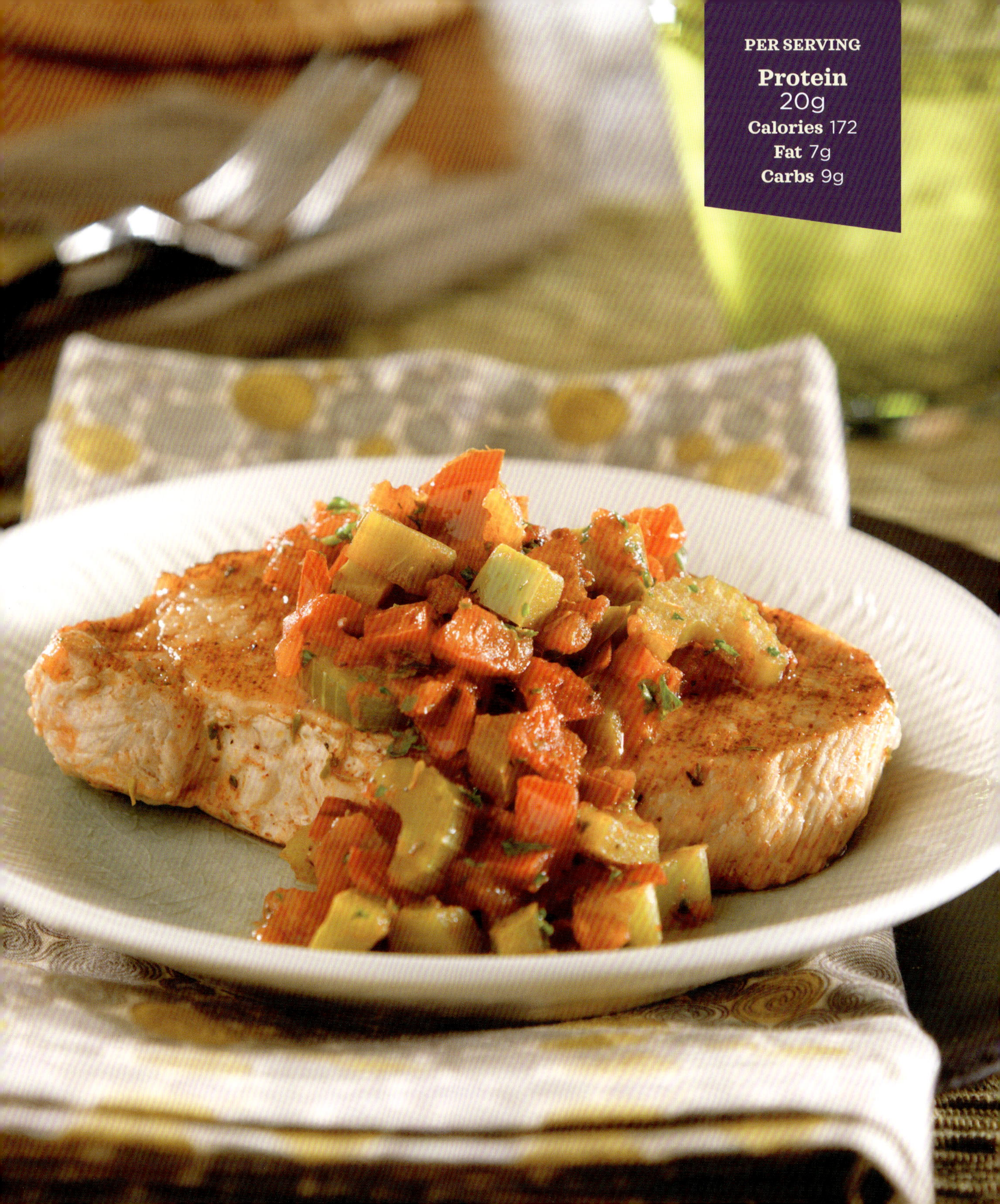
PER SERVING
Protein
20g
Calories 172
Fat 7g
Carbs 9g

Stuffed Eggplant

MAKES 4 SERVINGS

- **2 eggplants (8 to 12 ounces each), halved lengthwise**
- **1 teaspoon salt**
- **1½ teaspoons minced garlic**
- **1 teaspoon black pepper**
- **1 pound boneless beef sirloin steak, trimmed and cut into ¼-inch strips**
- **2 cups sliced red and green bell peppers**
- **2 cups sliced mushrooms**
- **¼ cup water**
- **Paprika (optional)**
- **Chopped fresh parsley (optional)**

1. Preheat oven to 450°F. Spray large baking dish with nonstick cooking spray.

2. Place eggplant cut sides up in prepared baking dish; pierce each half with fork about 8 times. Sprinkle each half with ¼ teaspoon salt. Cover with foil and bake 45 minutes.

3. Meanwhile, spray large nonstick skillet with cooking spray. Add garlic and black pepper; cook and stir over medium heat 2 minutes. Add beef; cook and stir 5 minutes. Add bell peppers; cook 5 minutes. Add mushrooms; cook 5 minutes, stirring occasionally. Stir in water. Remove from heat; cover and let stand until ready to use.

4. Remove eggplant from oven, set aside to cool 5 minutes. Mash cooked eggplant centers with fork, being careful not to break shells. Top each half with one fourth of beef mixture; stir beef mixture into mashed eggplant.

5. Cover with foil; bake 15 minutes. Garnish with paprika and parsley.

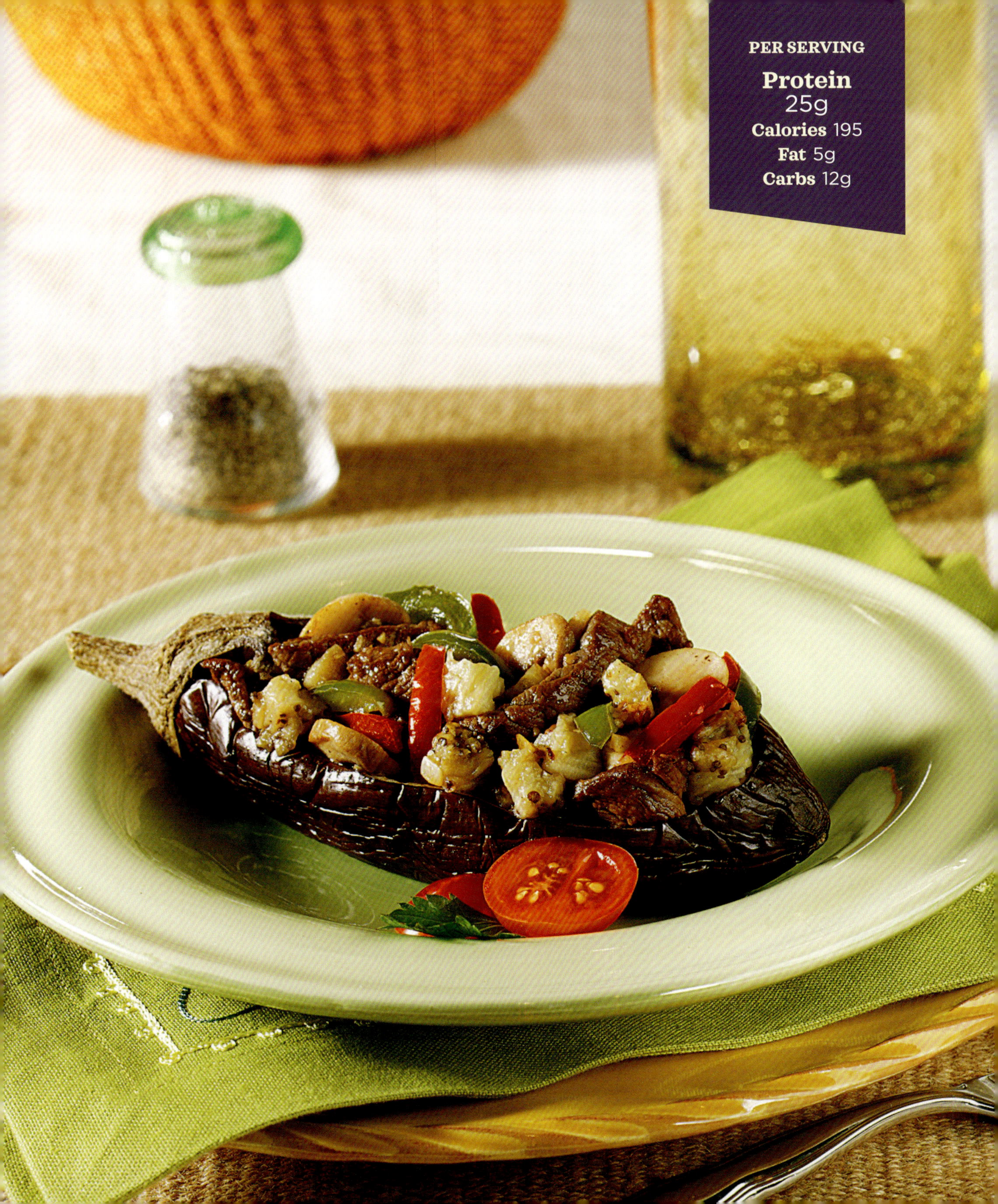
PER SERVING
Protein
25g
Calories 195
Fat 5g
Carbs 12g

Asian Peppercorn Beef

MAKES 4 SERVINGS

- **2 teaspoons whole black and pink peppercorns***
- **2 teaspoons coriander seeds**
- **1 tablespoon peanut or canola oil**
- **1 boneless beef top sirloin steak, about 1¼ inches thick (1¼ pounds)**
- **2 teaspoons dark sesame oil**
- **½ cup thinly sliced shallots or sweet onion**
- **½ cup beef broth**
- **2 tablespoons soy sauce**
- **1 tablespoon dry sherry**
- **2 tablespoons thinly sliced green onion or chopped fresh cilantro**

***Or substitute all black peppercorns.*

1 Combine peppercorns and coriander seeds in small resealable food storage bag. Seal bag; coarsely crush spices with meat mallet or bottom of heavy saucepan.

2 Brush peanut oil over both sides of steak; sprinkle with peppercorn mixture, pressing lightly to adhere.

3 Heat large skillet over medium-high heat. Add steak; cook 4 minutes without moving or until seared on bottom. Reduce heat to medium; turn steak and cook 3 to 4 minutes for medium rare or to desired doneness. Remove steak to cutting board; tent with foil and let stand while preparing sauce.

4 Add sesame oil to skillet; heat over medium heat. Add shallots; cook and stir 3 minutes. Add broth, soy sauce and sherry; cook 5 minutes.

5 Cut steak into thin slices; top with sauce and green onion.

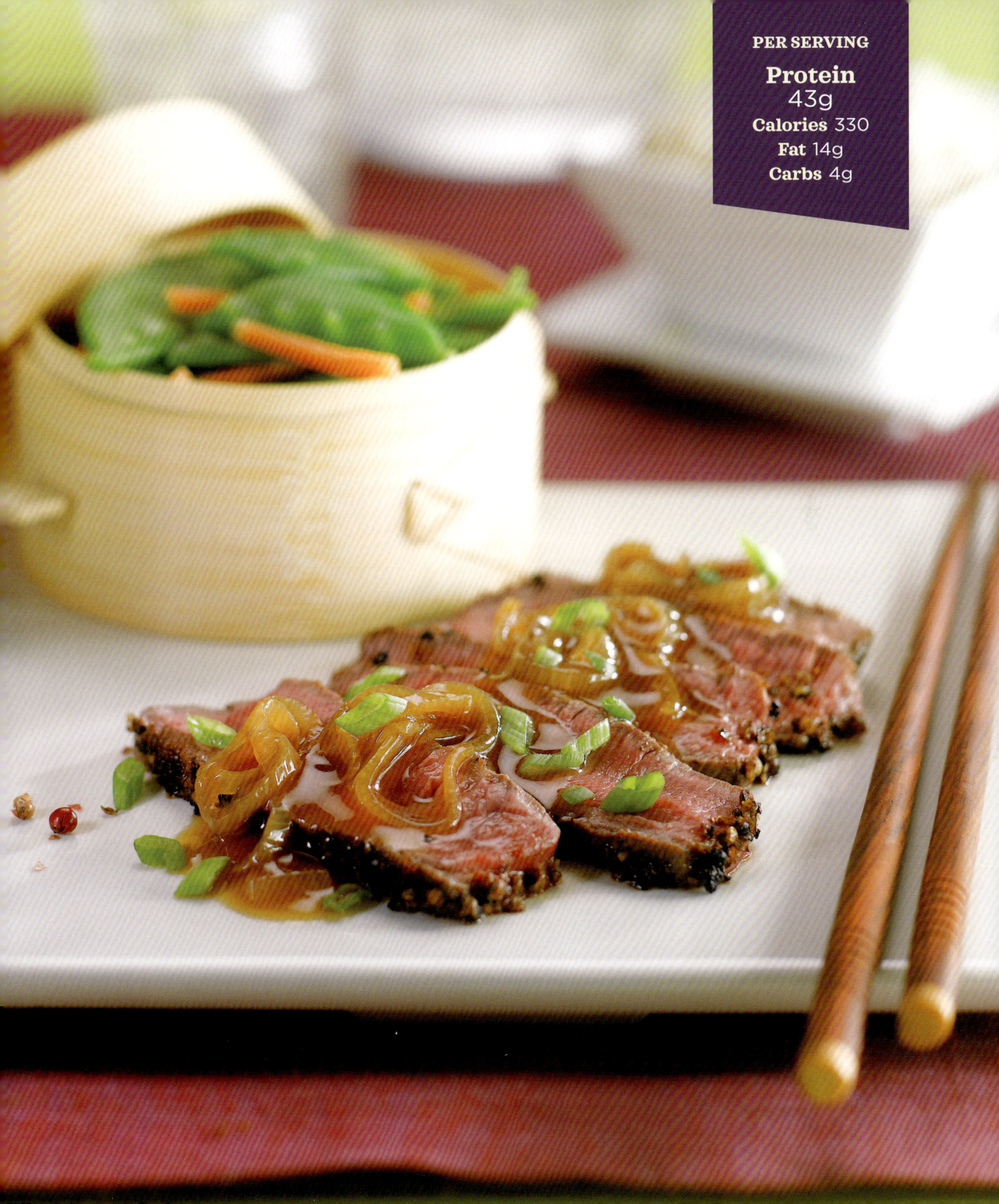
PER SERVING
Protein 43g
Calories 330
Fat 14g
Carbs 4g

Pork Curry over Cauliflower Couscous

MAKES 6 SERVINGS

- 3 tablespoons olive oil, divided
- 2 tablespoons mild curry powder
- 2 teaspoons minced garlic
- 1½ pounds boneless pork (shoulder, loin or chops), cut into 1-inch pieces
- 1 red and/or green bell pepper, diced
- 1 tablespoon cider vinegar
- ½ teaspoon salt
- 2 cups water
- 1 large head cauliflower
- Fresh cilantro sprigs (optional)

1. Heat 2 tablespoons oil in large saucepan over medium heat. Add curry powder and garlic; cook and stir 1 to 2 minutes or until garlic is golden brown.
2. Add pork; cook and stir 5 to 7 minutes or until barely pink in center. Add bell pepper and vinegar; cook and stir 3 minutes or until bell pepper is tender. Sprinkle with salt.
3. Stir in water; bring to a boil. Reduce heat to low; simmer 30 to 45 minutes or until liquid is reduced and pork is tender, stirring occasionally and adding additional water as needed.
4. Meanwhile, trim and core cauliflower; cut into large chunks. Place in food processor; pulse until cauliflower is in small uniform pieces about the size of cooked couscous. (Do not purée.)
5. Heat remaining 1 tablespoon oil in large nonstick skillet over medium heat. Add cauliflower; cook and stir 5 minutes or just until crisp-tender. Serve pork over cauliflower; garnish with cilantro.

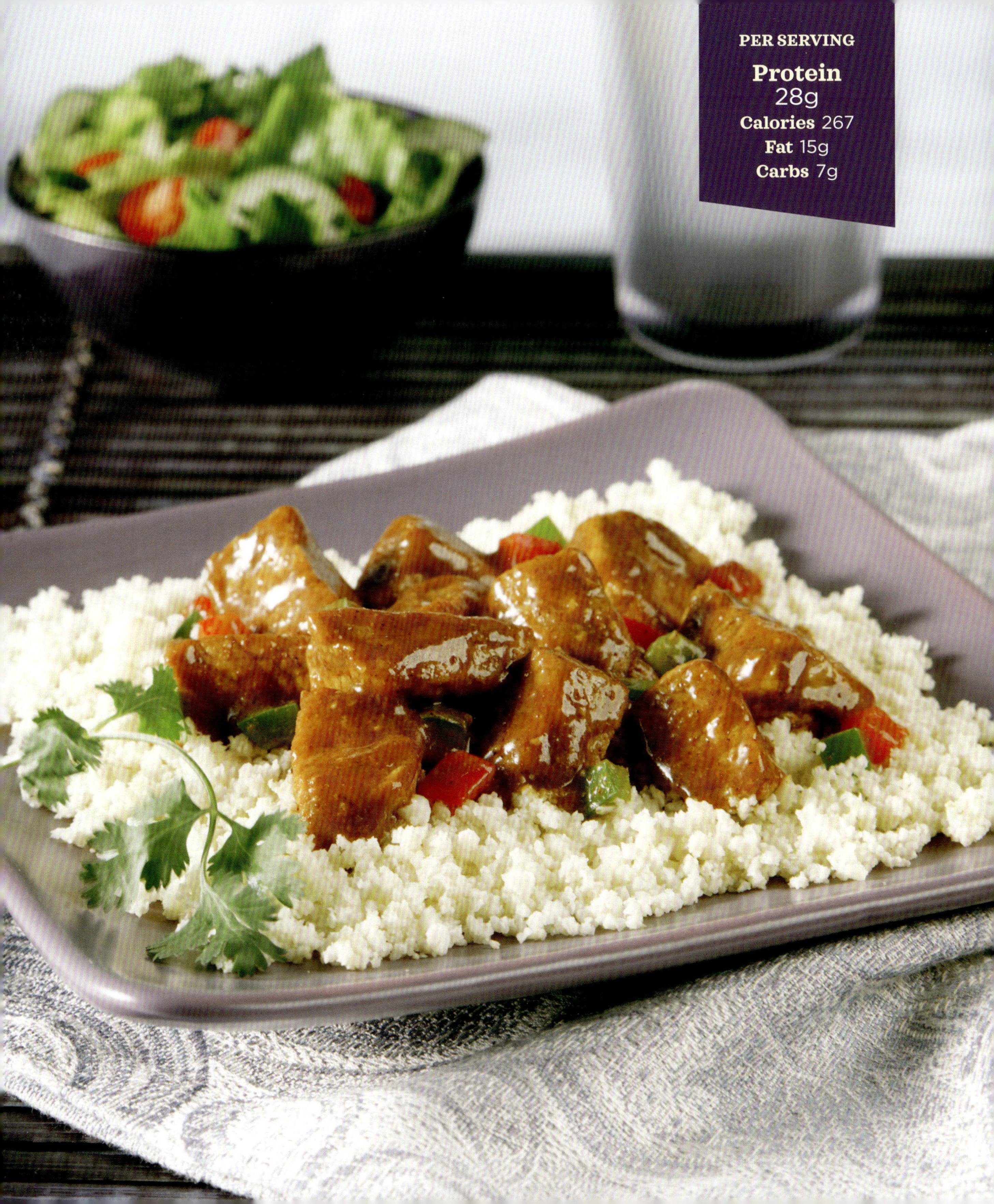
PER SERVING
Protein
28g
Calories 267
Fat 15g
Carbs 7g

Grilled Strip Steaks with Chimichurri

MAKES 4 SERVINGS

- **4 bone-in strip steaks (8 ounces each), about 1 inch thick**
- **¾ teaspoon salt**
- **¾ teaspoon ground cumin**
- **¼ teaspoon black pepper**
- **Chimichurri (recipe follows)**

1 Prepare grill for direct cooking over medium-high heat. Oil grill grate.

2 Prepare Chimichurri. Sprinkle both sides of steaks with salt, cumin and pepper.

3 Grill steaks, covered, 4 to 5 minutes per side for medium rare (135°F) or to desired doneness. Serve with Chimichurri.

Chimichurri

MAKES ABOUT 1 CUP

- **½ cup packed fresh basil**
- **⅓ cup olive oil**
- **¼ cup packed fresh parsley**
- **2 tablespoons packed fresh cilantro**
- **2 tablespoons lemon juice**
- **1 clove garlic**
- **½ teaspoon salt**
- **½ teaspoon grated orange peel**
- **¼ teaspoon ground coriander**
- **⅛ teaspoon black pepper**

Combine basil, oil, parsley, cilantro, lemon juice, garlic, salt, orange peel, coriander and pepper in food processor or blender; process until almost smooth.

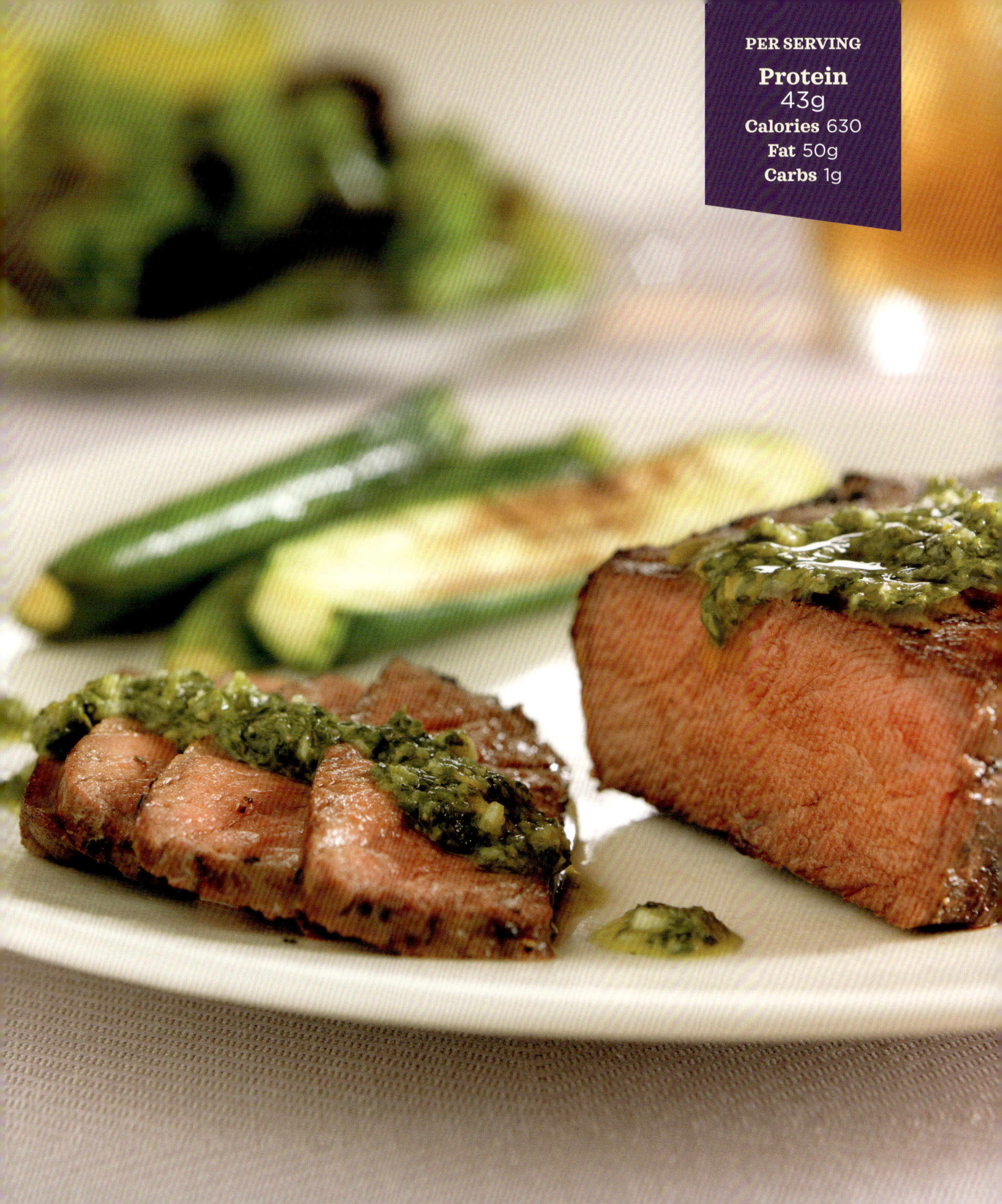
PER SERVING
Protein
43g
Calories 630
Fat 50g
Carbs 1g

Pork and Plum Kabobs

MAKES 4 SERVINGS

- **12 ounces boneless pork loin chops (1 inch thick), trimmed and cut into 1-inch pieces**
- **1½ teaspoons ground cumin**
- **½ teaspoon ground cinnamon**
- **¼ teaspoon salt**
- **¼ teaspoon garlic powder**
- **¼ teaspoon ground red pepper**
- **¼ cup sliced green onion**
- **¼ cup raspberry fruit spread**
- **1 tablespoon orange juice**
- **3 plums or nectarines, pitted and cut into wedges**

1 Place pork in large resealable food storage bag. Combine cumin, cinnamon, salt, garlic powder and red pepper in small bowl; mix well. Add to pork; seal bag and shake to coat.

2 Combine green onion, fruit spread and orange juice in medium bowl; mix well.

3 Prepare grill for direct cooking over medium heat. Alternately thread pork and plum wedges onto eight skewers.*

4 Grill kabobs 6 to 7 minutes per side or until pork is barely pink in center (145°F). Brush frequently with raspberry mixture during last 5 minutes of grilling.

**If using wooden skewers, soak in cold water 20 to 30 minutes to prevent burning.*

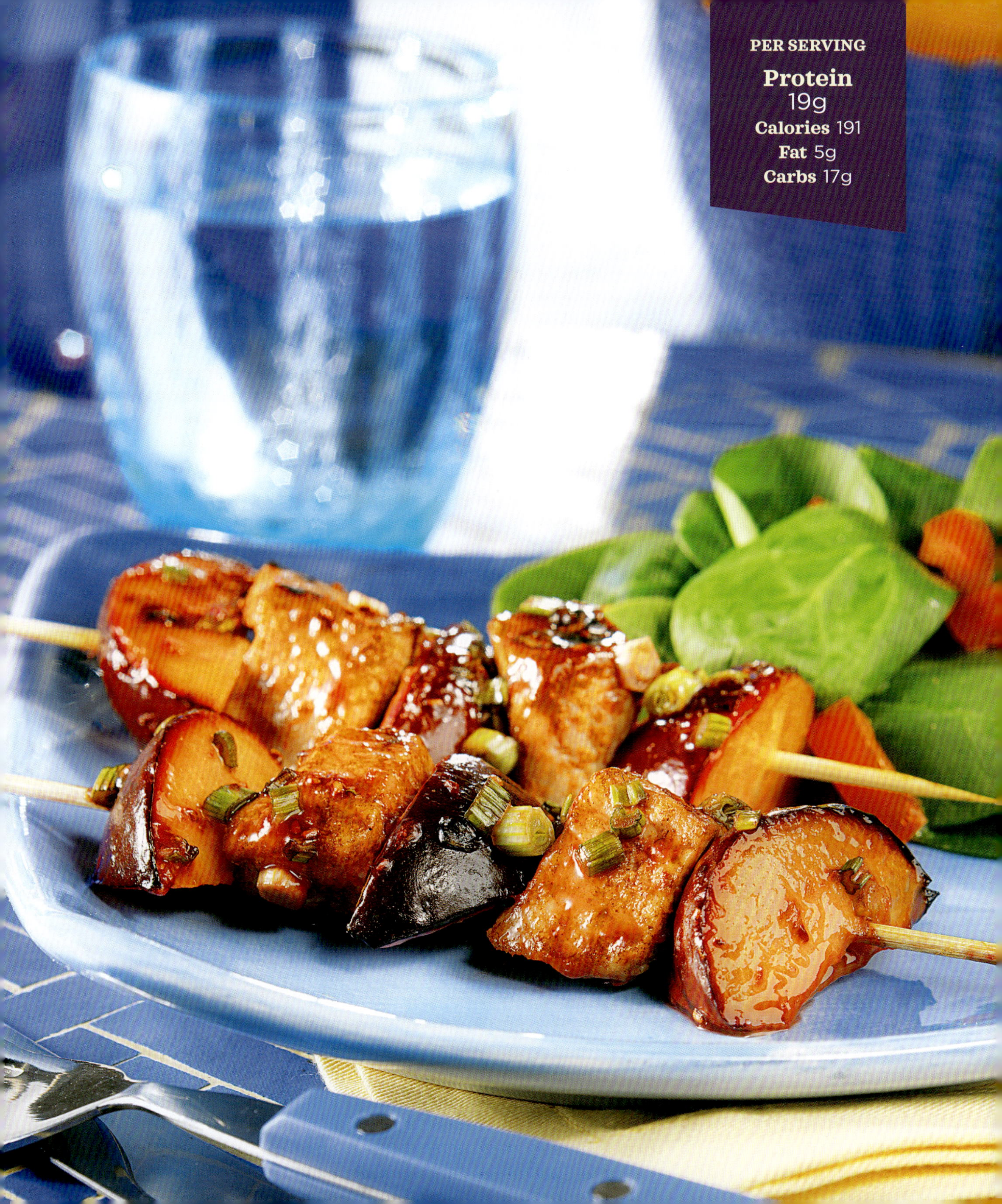
PER SERVING
Protein
19g
Calories 191
Fat 5g
Carbs 17g

Blue Cheese-Stuffed Sirloin Patties

MAKES 4 SERVINGS

- **1½ pounds ground beef sirloin**
- **½ cup (2 ounces) shredded sharp Cheddar cheese**
- **¼ cup crumbled blue cheese**
- **¼ cup finely chopped fresh parsley**
- **2 teaspoons Dijon mustard**
- **1 clove garlic, minced**
- **1 teaspoon Worcestershire sauce**
- **¼ teaspoon salt**
- **2 teaspoons olive oil**
- **1 medium red bell pepper, cut into thin strips**

1. Shape beef into eight patties, about 4 inches in diameter and ¼ inch thick.

2. Combine Cheddar, blue cheese, parsley, mustard, garlic, Worcestershire sauce and ¼ teaspoon salt in small bowl; mix well.

3. Mound one fourth of cheese mixture on each of four patties (about 3 tablespoons per patty). Top with remaining four patties; pinch edges of patties to seal.

4. Heat oil in large skillet over medium-high heat. Add bell pepper; cook and stir 5 minutes or until edges of peppers begin to brown. Sprinkle with salt. Remove to plate; tent with foil to keep warm.

5. Add beef patties to skillet; cook 5 minutes. Turn patties; top with bell peppers. Cook about 4 minutes for medium (140° to 145°F) or to desired doneness.

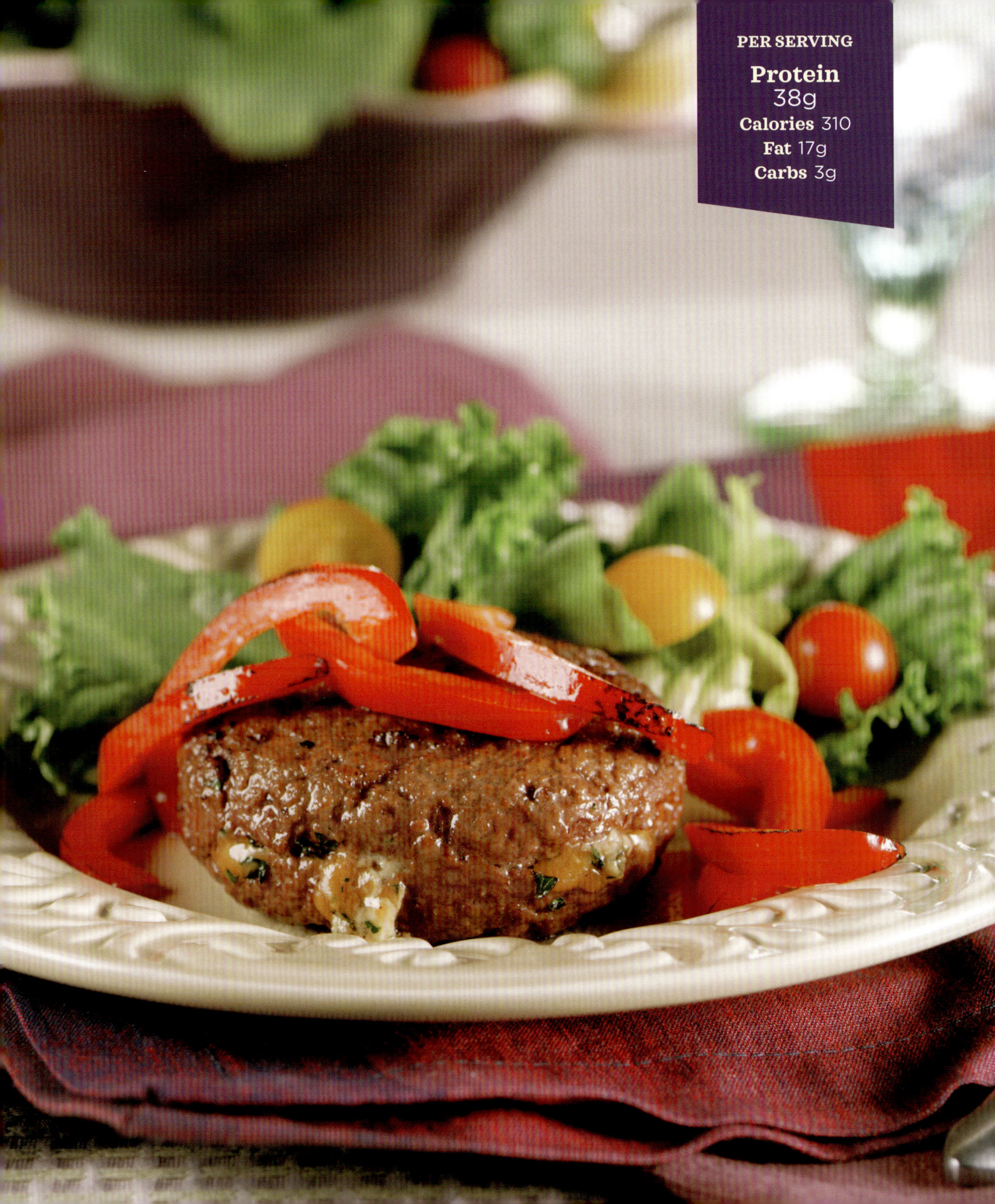
PER SERVING
Protein
38g
Calories 310
Fat 17g
Carbs 3g

PER SERVING
Protein
26g
Calories 180
Fat 5g
Carbs 4g

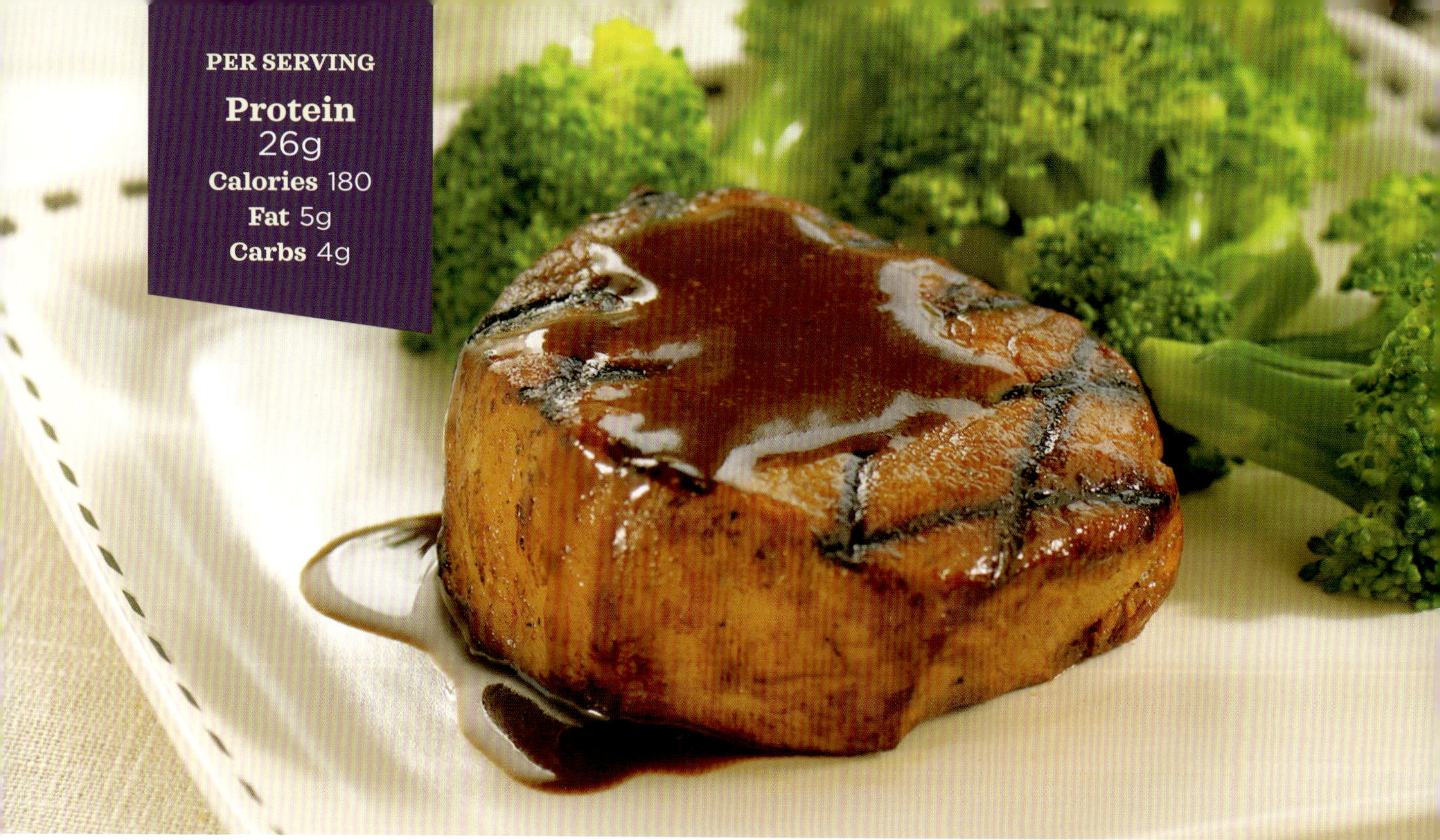

Balsamic Grilled Pork Chops

MAKES 2 SERVINGS

- 2 boneless pork chops, trimmed (about 4 ounces each)
- 2 tablespoons balsamic vinegar
- 2 tablespoons soy sauce
- 1 teaspoon Dijon mustard
- ⅛ teaspoon red pepper flakes

1. Place pork in large resealable food storage bag. Combine vinegar, soy sauce, mustard and red pepper flakes in small bowl; mix well.

2. Reserve 1 tablespoon marinade in small bowl; set aside. Pour remaining marinade over pork; seal bag and turn to coat. Marinate in refrigerator 2 hours or up to 24 hours.

3. Spray grill pan with nonstick cooking spray; heat over medium-high heat. Remove pork from marinade; discard marinade.

4. Cook pork 4 minutes per side or until barely pink in center (145°F). Top with reserved 1 tablespoon marinade.

PER SERVING
Protein
27g
Calories 214
Fat 9g
Carbs 6g

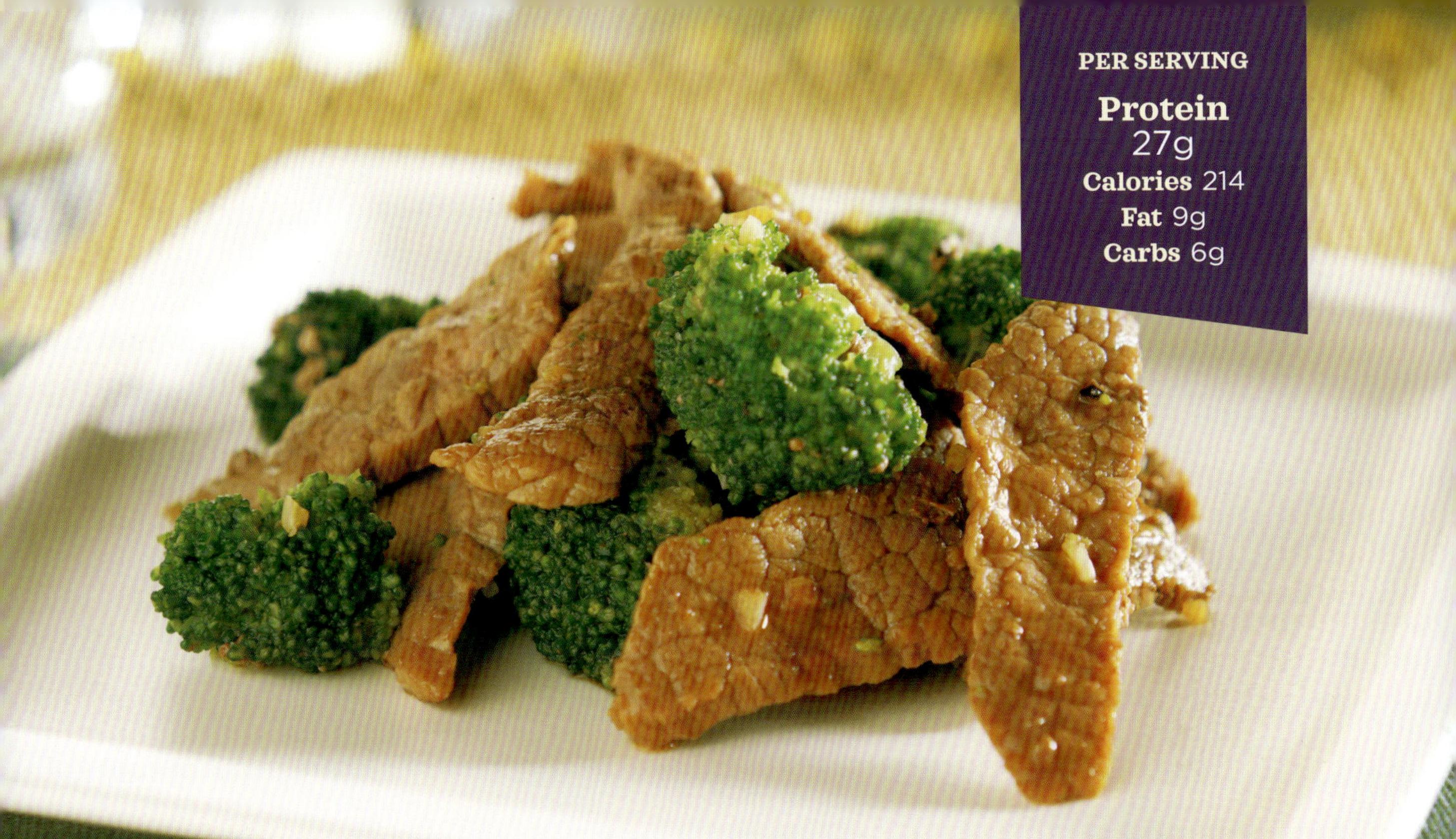

Garlic Beef

MAKES 4 SERVINGS

- 1 teaspoon dark sesame oil
- 1 pound beef eye of round, trimmed, cut into thin strips
- 1 package (10 ounces) frozen chopped broccoli
- 1 tablespoon minced garlic
- 1 tablespoon soy sauce
- ¼ teaspoon black pepper

Heat oil in large skillet over high heat. Add beef, broccoli, garlic, soy sauce and pepper; cook 15 minutes or until beef is tender, stirring occasionally.

Beef and Pepper Kabobs

MAKES 4 SERVINGS

- **8 ounces sirloin steak, trimmed**
- **2 teaspoons reduced-sodium soy sauce**
- **2 teaspoons red wine vinegar**
- **1½ teaspoons Dijon mustard**
- **1 teaspoon olive oil**
- **1 clove garlic, minced**
- **⅛ teaspoon black pepper**
- **2 bell peppers (any color), each cut into 12 pieces**
- **1 tablespoon chicken or vegetable broth**
- **4 large green onions**

1. Cut steak into 16 (¼-inch) strips; place in medium bowl. Whisk soy sauce, vinegar, mustard, oil, garlic and black pepper in small bowl until well blended.
2. Add half of mixture to steak; stir to coat. Cover and refrigerate 2 to 3 hours, stirring occasionally. Cover and refrigerate remaining marinade until ready to use.
3. Prepare grill for direct cooking over medium-high heat. Thread bell pepper pieces onto four skewers.* Thread four beef strips onto each of four skewers.* Stir broth into reserved marinade.
4. Grill bell pepper skewers 5 to 7 minutes per side or until well browned and tender. Grill green onions 3 to 5 minutes or until well browned on both sides. Brush bell peppers and green onions lightly with marinade once during grilling.
5. Grill beef skewers 2 minutes per side, basting once per side with marinade. Coarsely chop green onions; sprinkle over beef and peppers.

**If using wooden skewers, soak in cold water 20 to 30 minutes to prevent burning.*

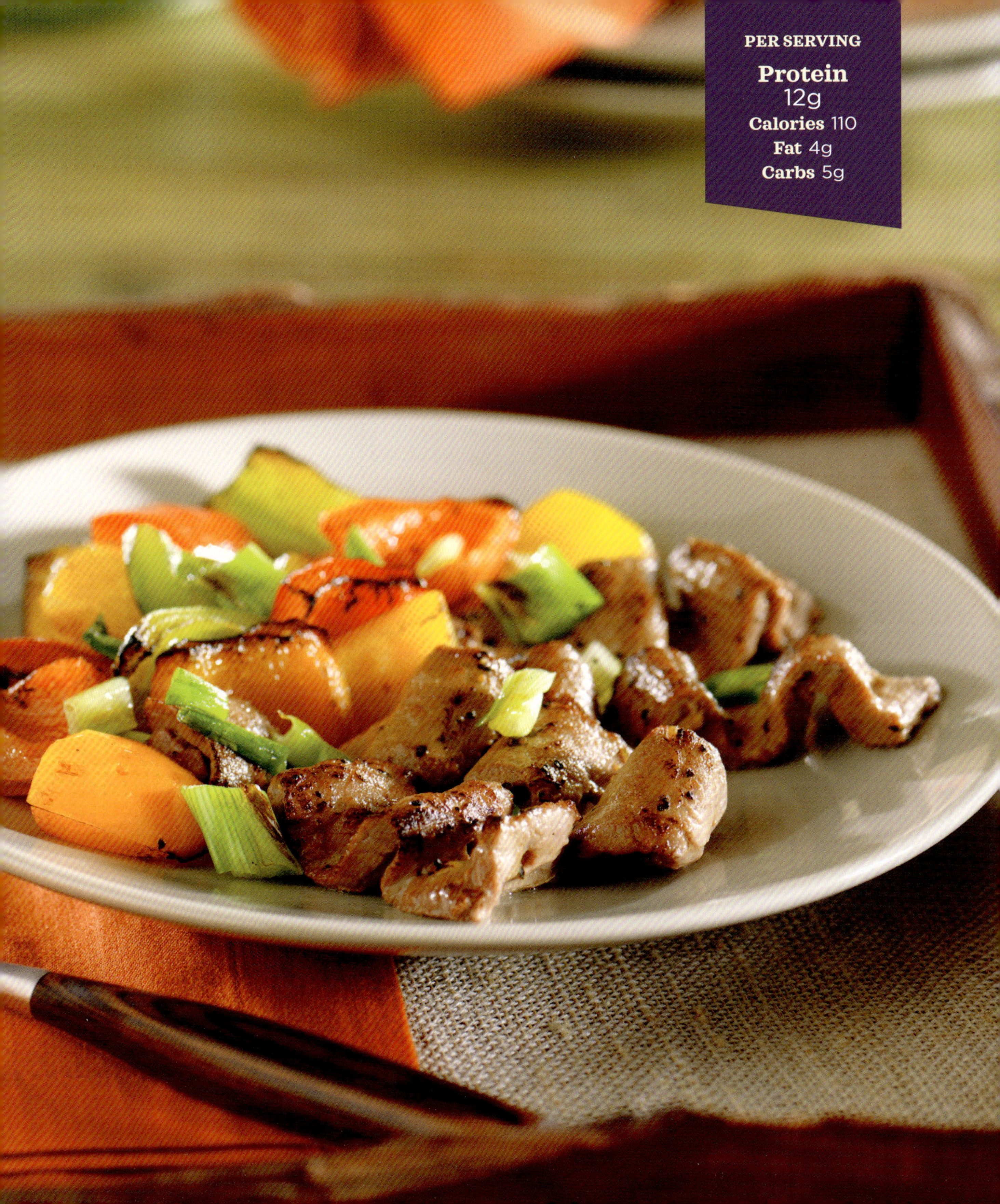

PER SERVING

Protein 12g

Calories 110

Fat 4g

Carbs 5g

Pork Tenderloin with Avocado-Tomatillo Salsa

MAKES 4 SERVINGS

Pork

- 1 tablespoon chili powder
- 1 teaspoon ground cumin
- 2 pounds pork tenderloin
- 2 teaspoons olive oil

Salsa

- 4 medium tomatillos, husked* and diced
- 1 ripe medium avocado, diced
- ¼ cup finely chopped red onion
- 2 jalapeño peppers, seeded and finely chopped
- 2 tablespoons lime juice
- 2 tablespoons chopped fresh cilantro
- 2 cloves garlic, minced
- ¼ teaspoon salt
- 8 lime wedges (optional)

***Remove the husk by pulling from the bottom to where it attaches at the stem. Wash before using.**

1 Preheat oven to 425°F. Line baking sheet with foil; spray foil with nonstick cooking spray. Combine chili powder and cumin in small bowl. Sprinkle all over pork, pressing to adhere.

2 Heat oil in large nonstick skillet over medium-high heat. Add pork; cook 3 minutes. Turn and cook 2 to 3 minutes or until well browned. Place on prepared baking sheet.

3 Roast pork 20 to 25 minutes or until barely pink in center (145°). Remove to cutting board; tent with foil and let stand 5 minutes before slicing.

4 Meanwhile, combine tomatillos, avocado, onion, jalapeños, lime juice, cilantro, garlic and salt in medium bowl; stir gently to blend.

5 Slice pork; serve with salsa and lime wedges, if desired.

Tip

Choose firm tomatillos with dry husks that are not too ragged. Store in a paper bag in the refrigerator for up to 1 month.

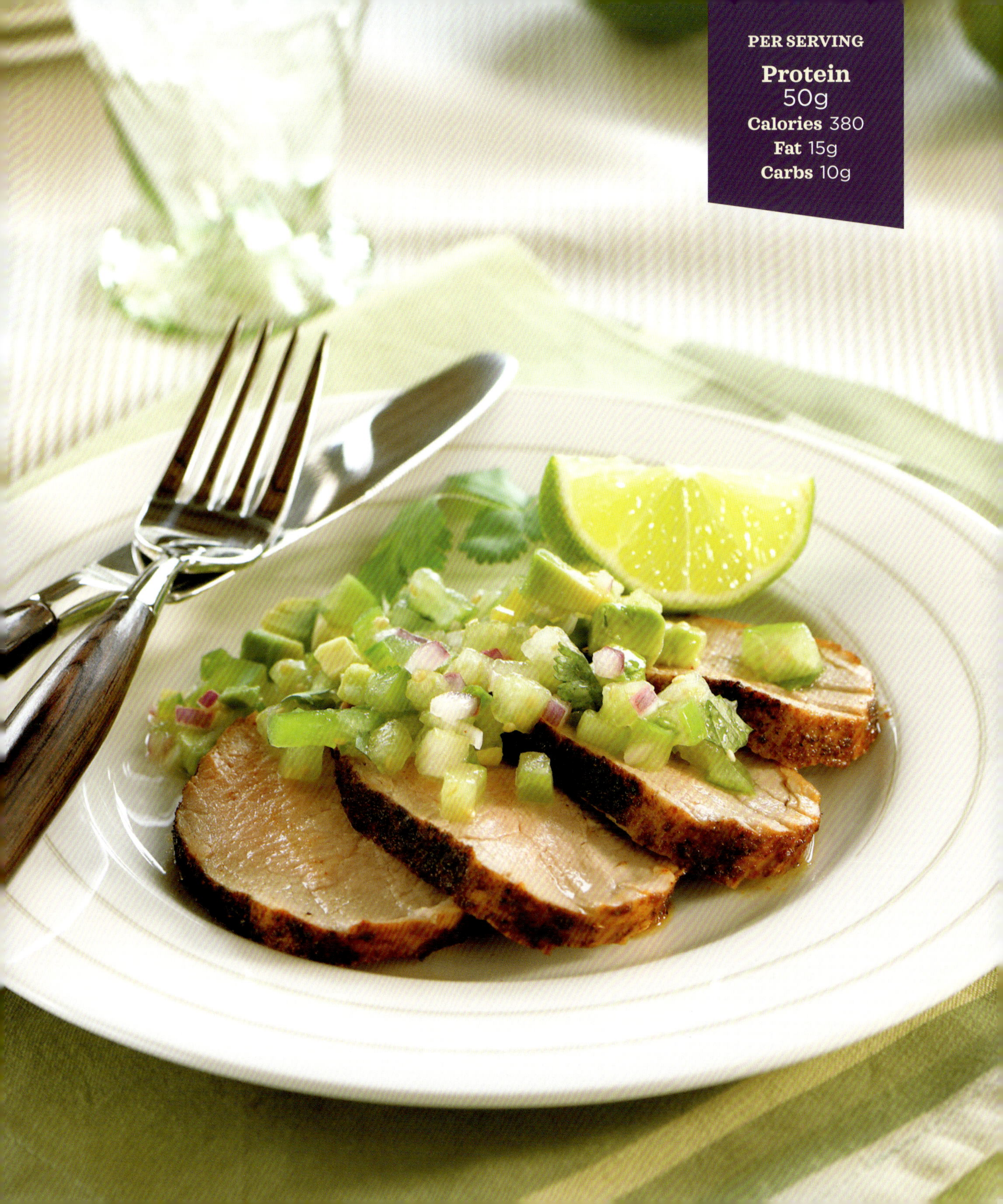

PER SERVING

Protein 50g
Calories 380
Fat 15g
Carbs 10g

Mini Meatloaves

MAKES 6 SERVINGS

- **3 tablespoons ketchup**
- **1 tablespoon balsamic vinegar**
- **1 tablespoon olive oil**
- **1½ cups finely chopped onion**
- **1½ cups finely chopped mushrooms**
- **1½ cups chopped baby spinach**
- **1½ pounds extra lean ground sirloin**
- **¾ cup old-fashioned oats**
- **2 egg whites**
- **½ teaspoon salt**
- **½ teaspoon black pepper**

1. Preheat oven to 375°F. Spray 6 mini (4¼×2½-inch) loaf pans with nonstick cooking spray.
2. Whisk ketchup and vinegar in small bowl until well blended; set aside.
3. Heat oil in large skillet over medium heat. Add onion, mushrooms and spinach; cook 8 minutes or until vegetables are tender, stirring frequently. Remove to large bowl; let stand until cool enough to handle.
4. Add beef, oats, egg whites, salt and pepper to vegetable mixture; stir until blended. Divide evenly among prepared pans; brush half of ketchup mixture evenly over loaves.
5. Bake 15 minutes. Brush with remaining ketchup mixture; bake 5 minutes or until cooked through (160°F).

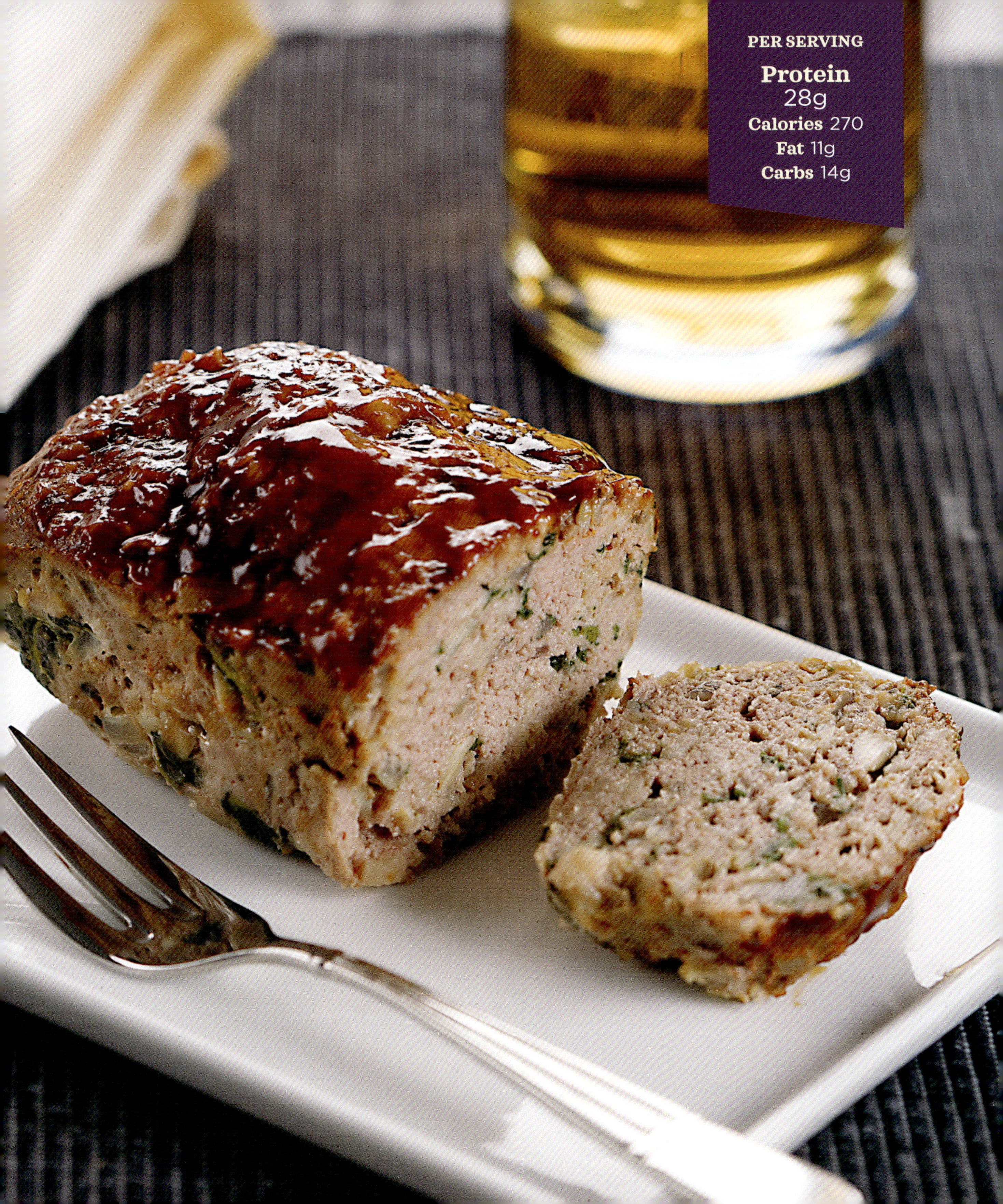
PER SERVING
Protein
28g
Calories 270
Fat 11g
Carbs 14g

Flank Steak with Italian Salsa

MAKES 6 SERVINGS

- 2 tablespoons olive oil
- 2 teaspoons balsamic vinegar
- 1 lean flank steak (1½ pounds)
- 1 tablespoon minced garlic
- ¾ teaspoon salt, divided
- ¾ teaspoon black pepper, divided
- 1 cup diced plum tomatoes
- ⅓ cup chopped pitted Kalamata olives
- 2 tablespoons chopped fresh basil

1. Whisk oil and vinegar in medium bowl until well blended. Place steak in shallow dish. Spread garlic over steak; sprinkle with ½ teaspoon salt and ½ teaspoon pepper. Spoon 2 tablespoons oil mixture over steak. Marinate in refrigerator at least 20 minutes or up to 2 hours.

2. Add tomatoes, olives, basil, remaining ¼ teaspoon salt and ¼ teaspoon pepper to remaining 2 teaspoons vinegar mixture in bowl; mix well.

3. Prepare grill for direct cooking over medium-high heat or preheat broiler. Remove steak from marinade; discard marinade. (Leave garlic on steak.)

4. Grill steak 5 to 6 minutes per side for medium rare (135°F) or to desired doneness. Remove to cutting board; tent with foil and let stand 5 minutes.

5. Cut steak into thin slices across the grain. Serve with tomato mixture.

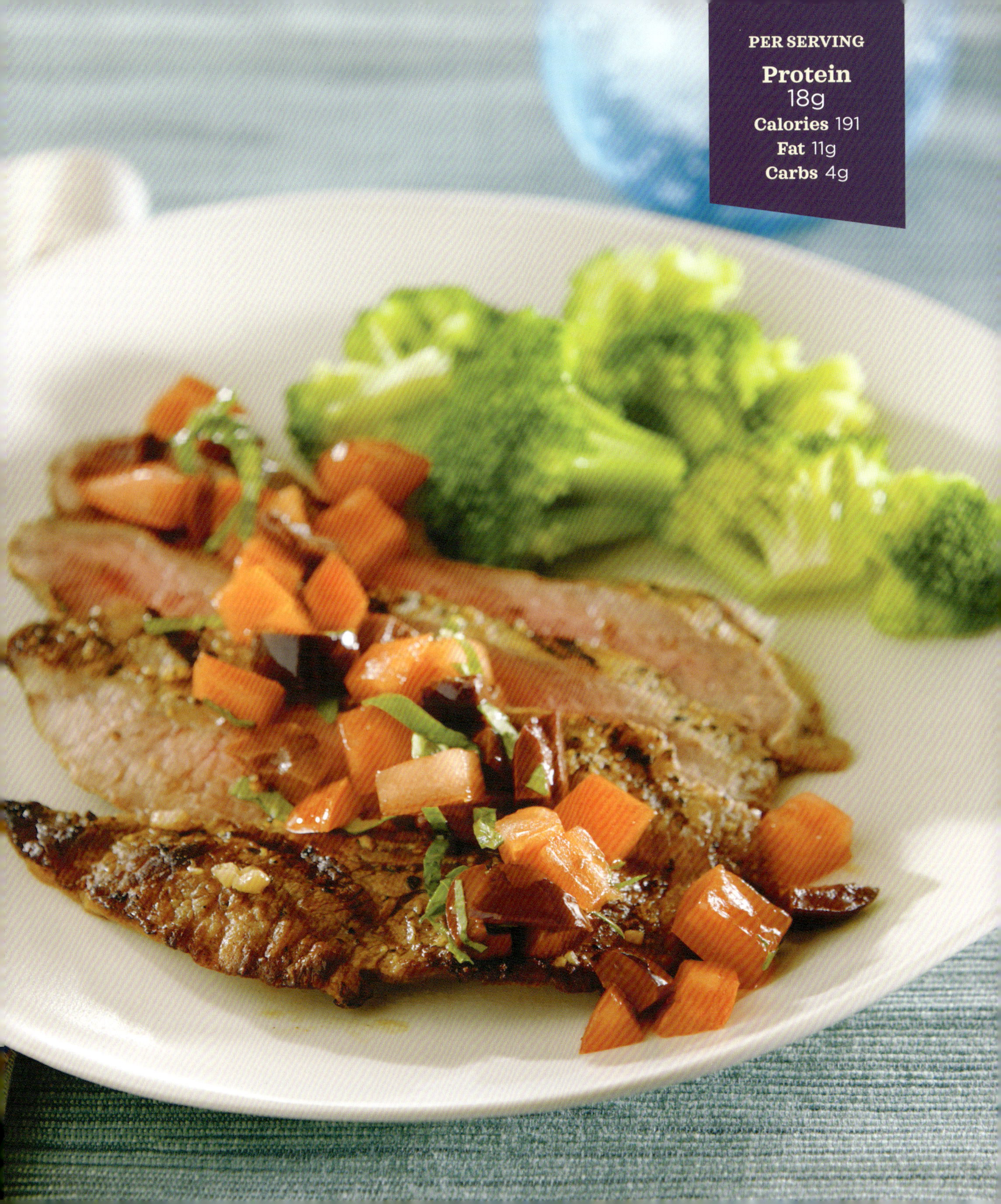
PER SERVING
Protein
18g
Calories 191
Fat 11g
Carbs 4g

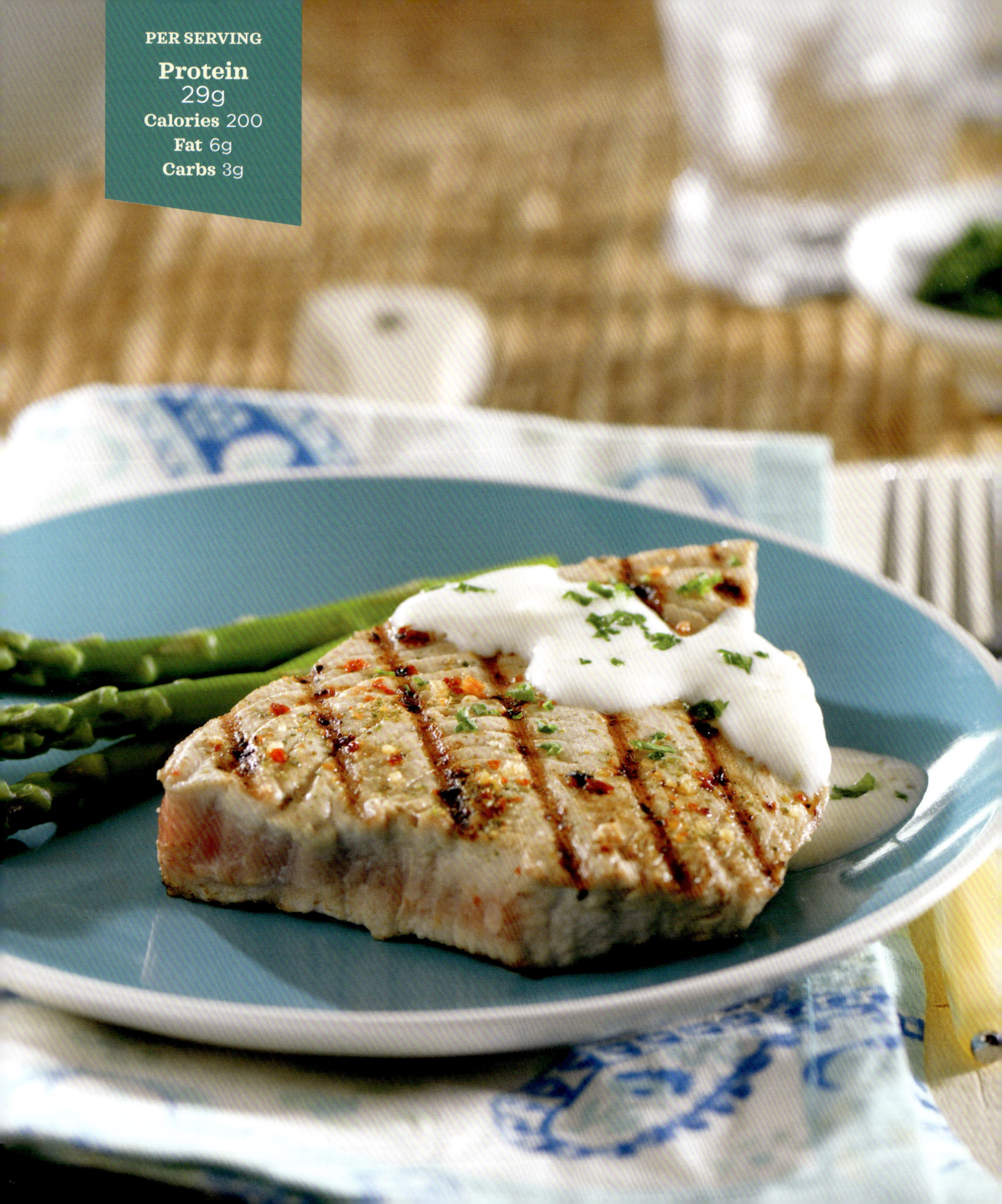
PER SERVING
Protein
29g
Calories 200
Fat 6g
Carbs 3g

SEAFOOD

Tuna with Spicy Horseradish Sauce

MAKES 4 SERVINGS

- **½ cup sour cream**
- **1 tablespoon water**
- **2 teaspoons prepared horseradish**
- **1 teaspoon Dijon mustard**
- **1 medium clove garlic, minced**
- **½ teaspoon dried rosemary**
- **½ teaspoon salt**
- **4 tuna steaks (4 ounces each)**
- **2 teaspoons steak seasoning blend**
- **2 tablespoons finely chopped green onion or parsley**

1 Combine sour cream, water, horseradish, mustard, garlic, rosemary and salt in small bowl; mix well.

2 Pat tuna dry. Sprinkle both sides of fish with steak seasoning blend, pressing gently to adhere.

3 Spray grill pan with nonstick cooking spray; heat over medium-high heat.

4 Cook fish 1½ minutes per side. (Do not overcook.) Sprinkle with green onion; serve with sauce.

Southwest Roasted Salmon and Corn

MAKES 2 SERVINGS

- 2 medium ears fresh corn, unhusked
- 1 salmon fillet (about 6 ounces), cut in half
- 1 tablespoon plus 1 teaspoon lime juice, divided
- 1 clove garlic, minced
- ½ teaspoon chili powder
- ¼ teaspoon ground cumin
- ¼ teaspoon dried oregano
- ⅛ teaspoon salt, divided
- ⅛ teaspoon black pepper
- 2 teaspoons margarine or butter, melted
- 2 teaspoons minced fresh cilantro

1 Pull back husks from each ear of corn, leaving husks attached. Discard silk. Bring husks back up over each ear. Soak corn in cold water 20 minutes.

2 Preheat oven to 400°F. Spray shallow baking dish with nonstick cooking spray. Place fish, skin side down, in prepared dish; pour 1 tablespoon lime juice over fish. Marinate at room temperature 15 minutes.

3 Combine garlic, chili powder, cumin, oregano, half of salt and pepper in small bowl; mix well. Pat fish dry with paper towel; rub with garlic mixture.

4 Remove corn from water; place directly on oven rack. Roast 10 minutes. Turn corn and place fish in baking dish next to corn. Roast 15 minutes or until corn is tender and fish begins to flake when tested with fork.

5 Combine margarine, cilantro, remaining 1 teaspoon lime juice and salt in small bowl; mix well. Remove husks; brush mixture over corn. Serve with fish.

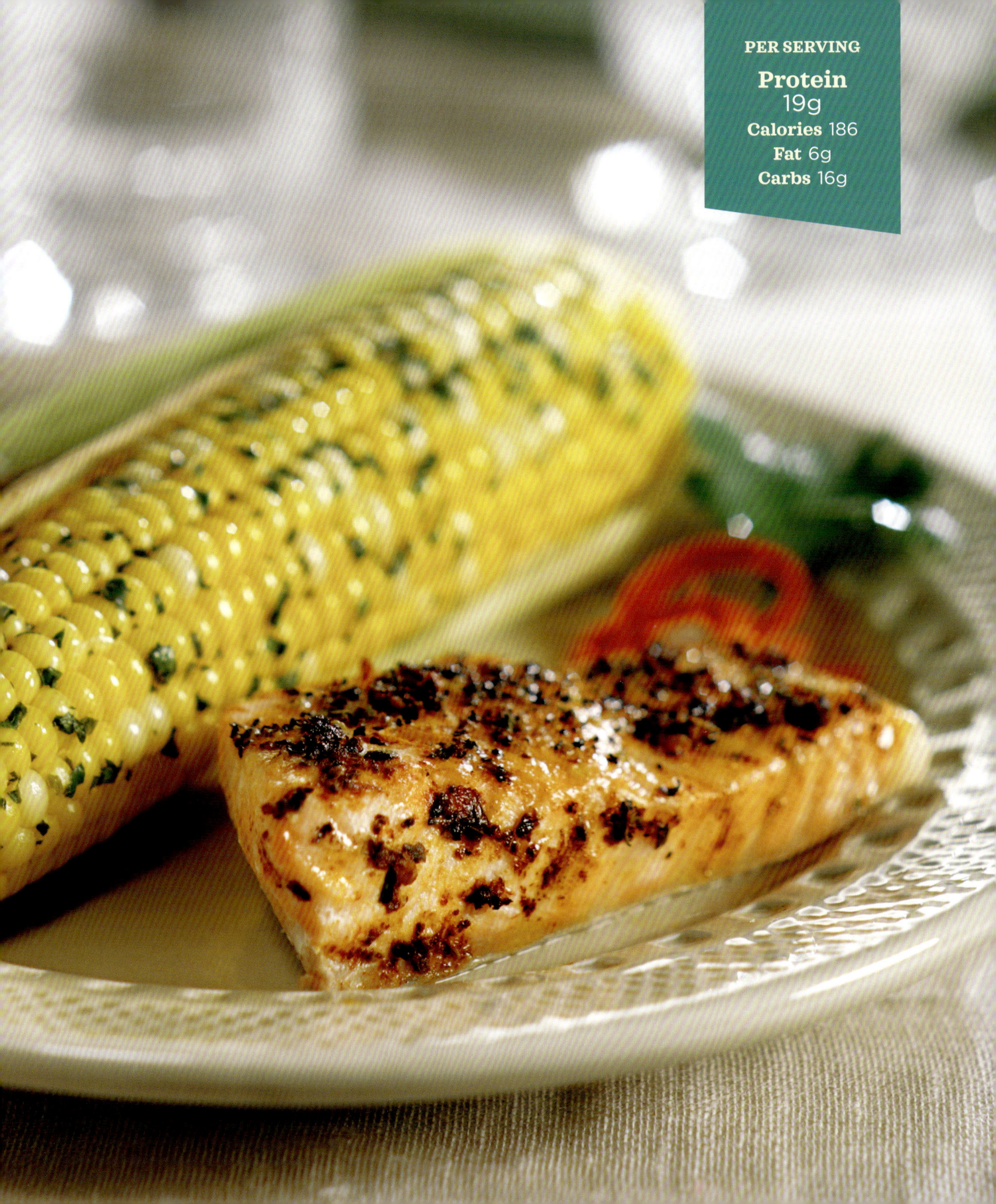
PER SERVING
Protein
19g
Calories 186
Fat 6g
Carbs 16g

Grilled Baja Burritos

MAKES 4 SERVINGS

- 6 tablespoons vegetable oil, divided
- 1 pound tilapia, snapper or halibut fillets
- 3 tablespoons lime juice, divided
- 2 teaspoons chili powder
- 1½ teaspoons lemon pepper
- 3 cups coleslaw mix
- ½ cup chopped fresh cilantro
- ¼ teaspoon salt
- ¼ teaspoon black pepper
- 4 (7-inch) flour tortillas
- Guacamole and pico de gallo (optional)
- Lime wedges (optional)

1 Prepare grill for direct cooking over medium-high heat or preheat broiler. Brush grill grate with 2 tablespoons oil.

2 Place fish in large resealable food storage bag. Combine 2 tablespoons oil, 1 tablespoon lime juice, chili powder and lemon pepper in small bowl; mix well. Drizzle over fish; seal bag and turn to coat. Marinate at room temperature 10 minutes.

3 Remove fish from marinade; discard marinade. Grill fish, covered, 3 to 4 minutes per side or until center is opaque. (To broil, place 4 inches from heat source; broil 3 to 5 minutes per side or until center is opaque.)

4 Combine coleslaw mix, remaining 2 tablespoons oil, 2 tablespoons lime juice, cilantro, salt and pepper in medium bowl; mix well.

5 Layer tortillas with fish, coleslaw mixture, guacamole and pico de gallo, if desired; roll up to enclose filling. Serve with additional pico de gallo and lime wedges, if desired.

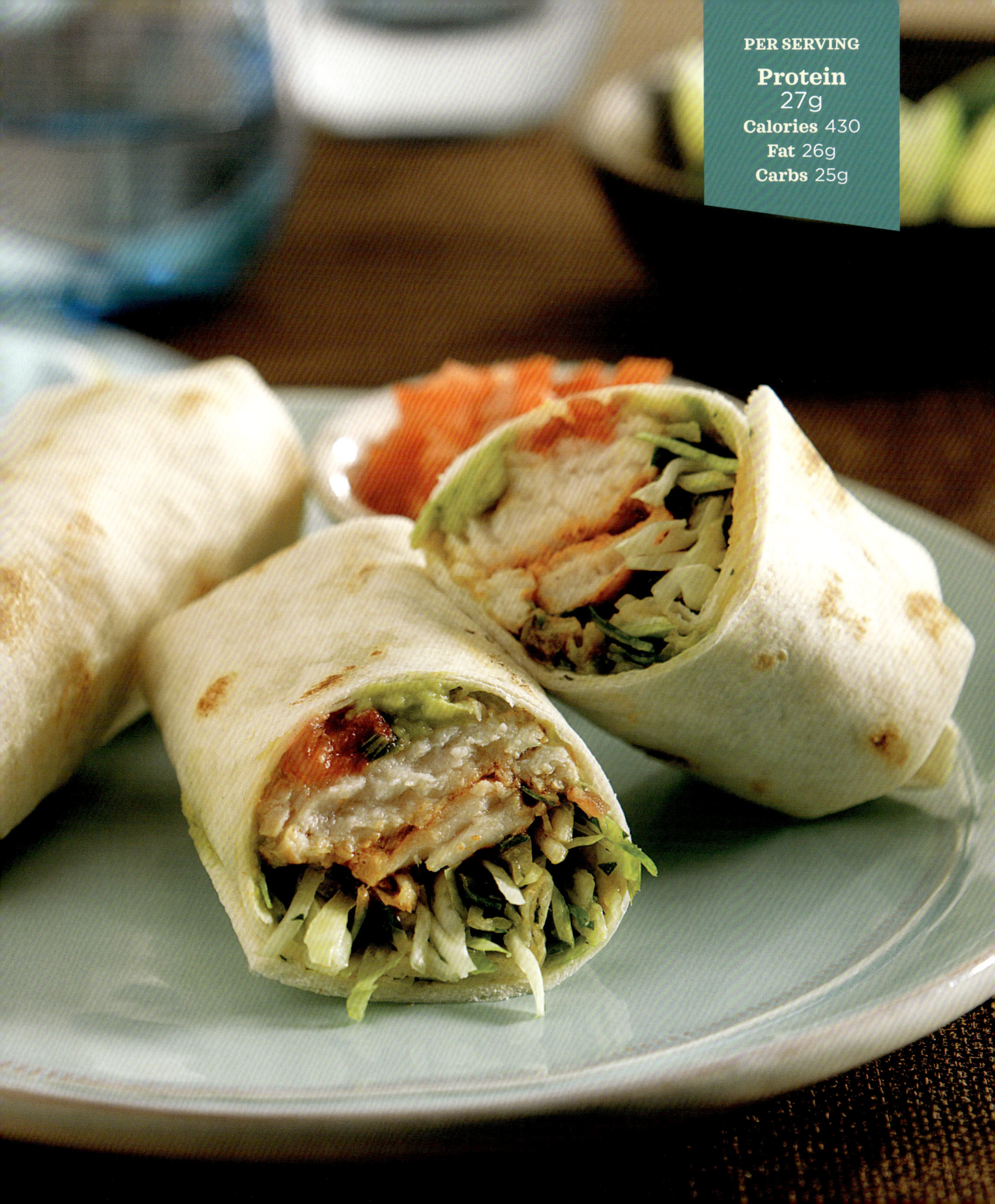

PER SERVING

Protein 27g
Calories 430
Fat 26g
Carbs 25g

PER SERVING
Protein
25g
Calories 410
Fat 14g
Carbs 45g

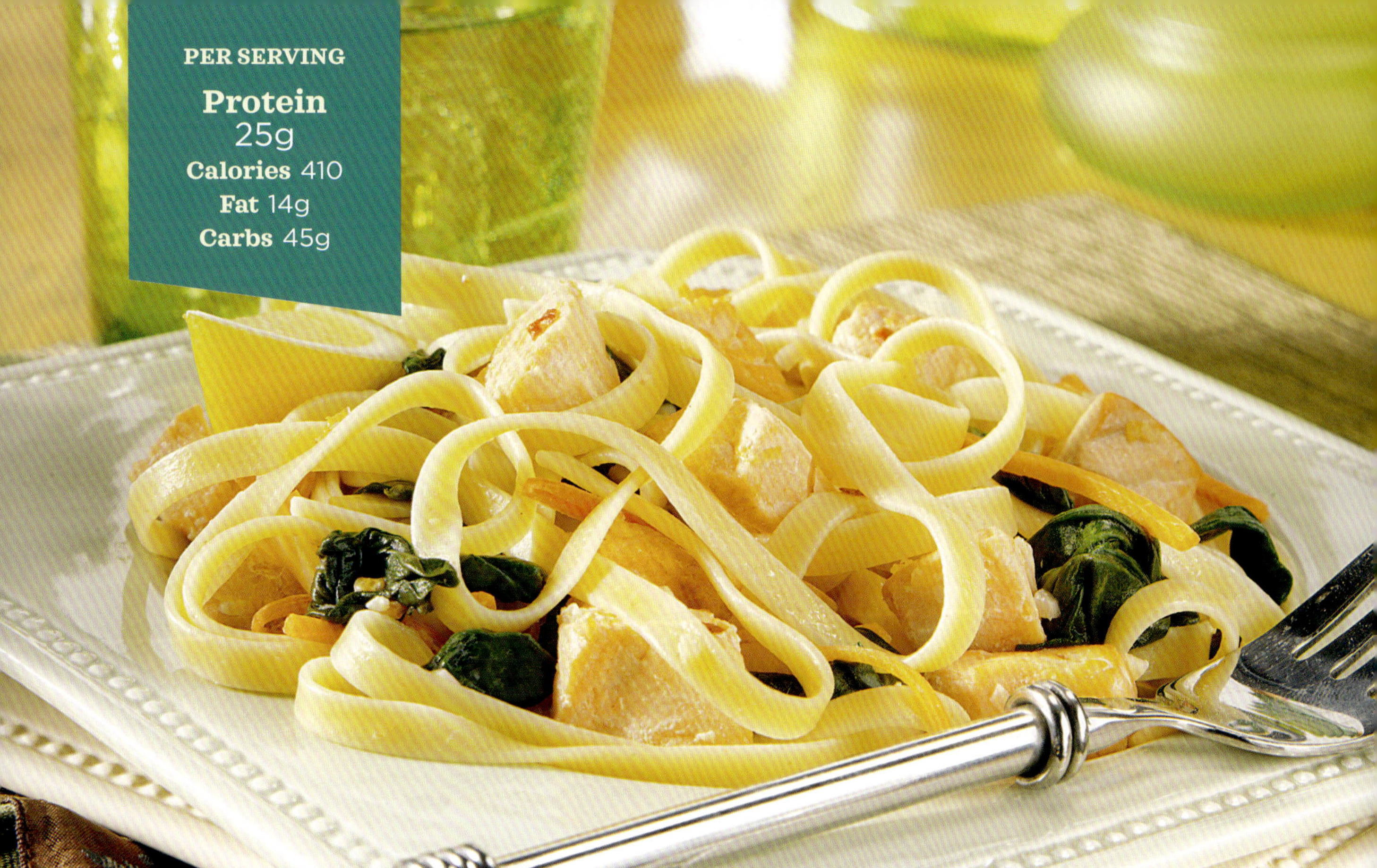

Lemon Salmon and Spinach Pasta

MAKES 4 SERVINGS

- 12 ounces salmon fillet
- 8 ounces uncooked fettuccine
- 4 teaspoons butter
- 1 teaspoon finely grated lemon peel
- ¼ teaspoon red pepper flakes
- 2 cloves garlic, minced
- 2 tablespoons lemon juice
- 3 cups baby spinach
- ½ cup shredded carrot

1 Pat fish dry with paper towel. Remove and discard skin; cut fish into ½-inch pieces.

2 Cook fettuccine according to package directions, omitting salt. Drain and return to saucepan.

3 Meanwhile, melt butter in large skillet over medium-high heat. Add fish, lemon peel, red pepper flakes and garlic; cook 4 to 6 minutes or until fish begins to flake when tested with fork. Gently stir in lemon juice.

4 Add fish mixture, spinach and carrot to hot cooked fettuccine; toss gently to combine. Serve immediately.

PER SERVING
Protein
35g
Calories 200
Fat 3g
Carbs 0g

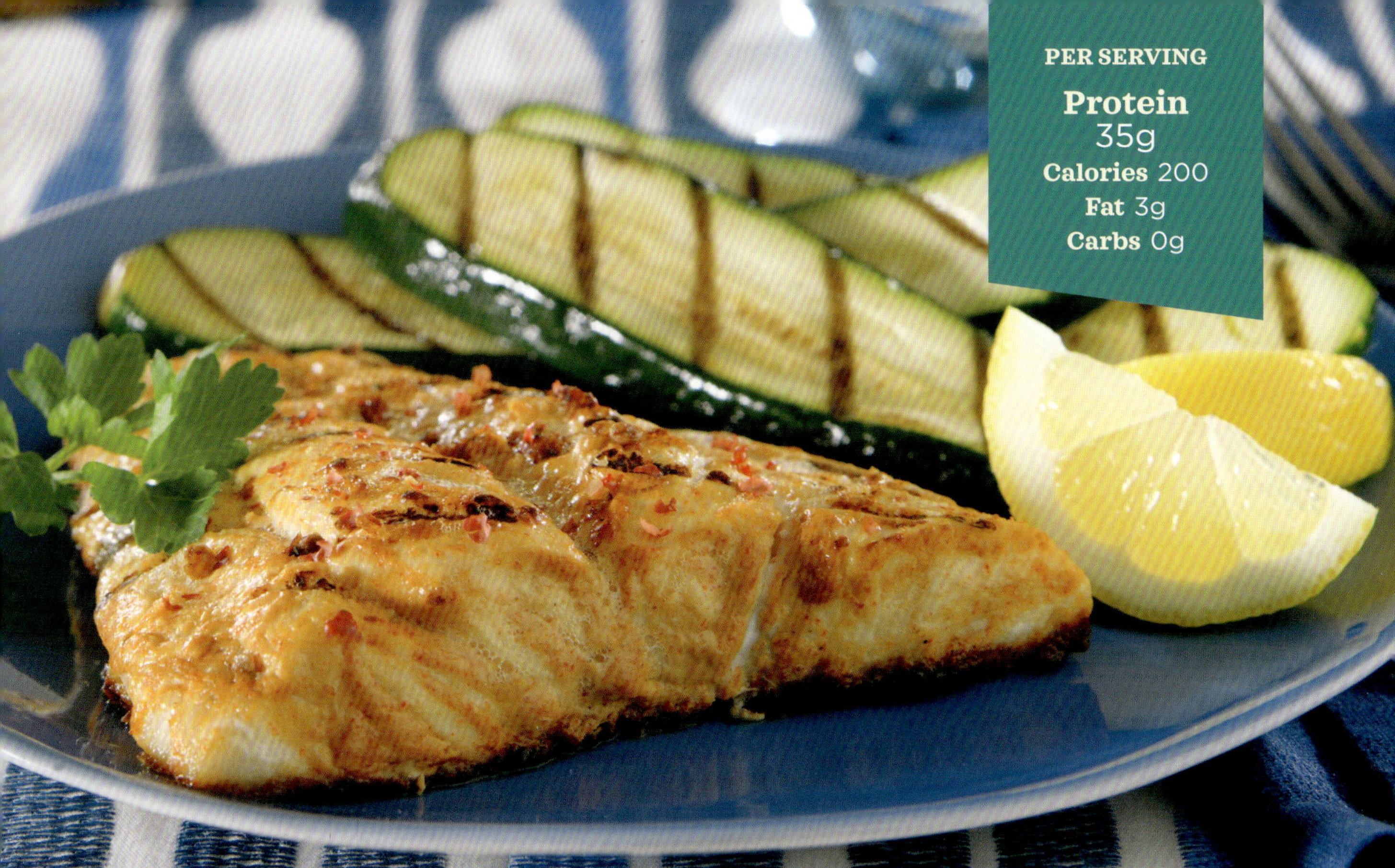

Mustard-Grilled Red Snapper

MAKES 4 SERVINGS

- ½ cup Dijon mustard
- 1 tablespoon red wine vinegar
- 1 teaspoon ground red pepper
- 4 red snapper fillets (about 6 ounces each)
- Fresh parsley sprigs (optional)

1 Prepare grill for direct cooking over medium-high heat. Spray grill grate with nonstick cooking spray.

2 Combine mustard, vinegar and red pepper in small bowl; mix well. Coat fish thoroughly with mustard mixture.

3 Grill fish, covered, 4 minutes per side or until fish begins to flake when tested with fork. Garnish with parsley.

Scallop and Artichoke Heart Casserole

MAKES 4 SERVINGS

- **1 package (9 ounces) frozen artichoke hearts, cooked and drained**
- **1 pound scallops**
- **1 teaspoon canola or vegetable oil**
- **¼ cup chopped red bell pepper**
- **¼ cup sliced green onions**
- **¼ cup all-purpose flour**
- **2 cups low-fat (1%) milk**
- **1 teaspoon dried tarragon**
- **¼ teaspoon salt**
- **¼ teaspoon white pepper**
- **1 tablespoon chopped fresh parsley**
- **Pinch paprika**

1. Preheat oven to 350°F. Spray 8-inch square baking dish with nonstick cooking spray.
2. Cut large artichokes lengthwise into halves; place in prepared baking dish.
3. Rinse scallops; pat dry with paper towel. If scallops are large, cut into halves. Arrange scallops over artichokes.
4. Heat oil in medium saucepan over medium-low heat. Add bell pepper and green onions; cook and stir 5 minutes or until vegetables are tender. Stir in flour until blended. Gradually stir in milk until smooth. Add tarragon, salt and white pepper; cook over medium heat 10 minutes or until sauce boils and thickens, stirring frequently. Pour sauce over scallops.
5. Bake, uncovered, 25 minutes or until casserole is bubbly and scallops are opaque. Sprinkle with parsley and paprika.

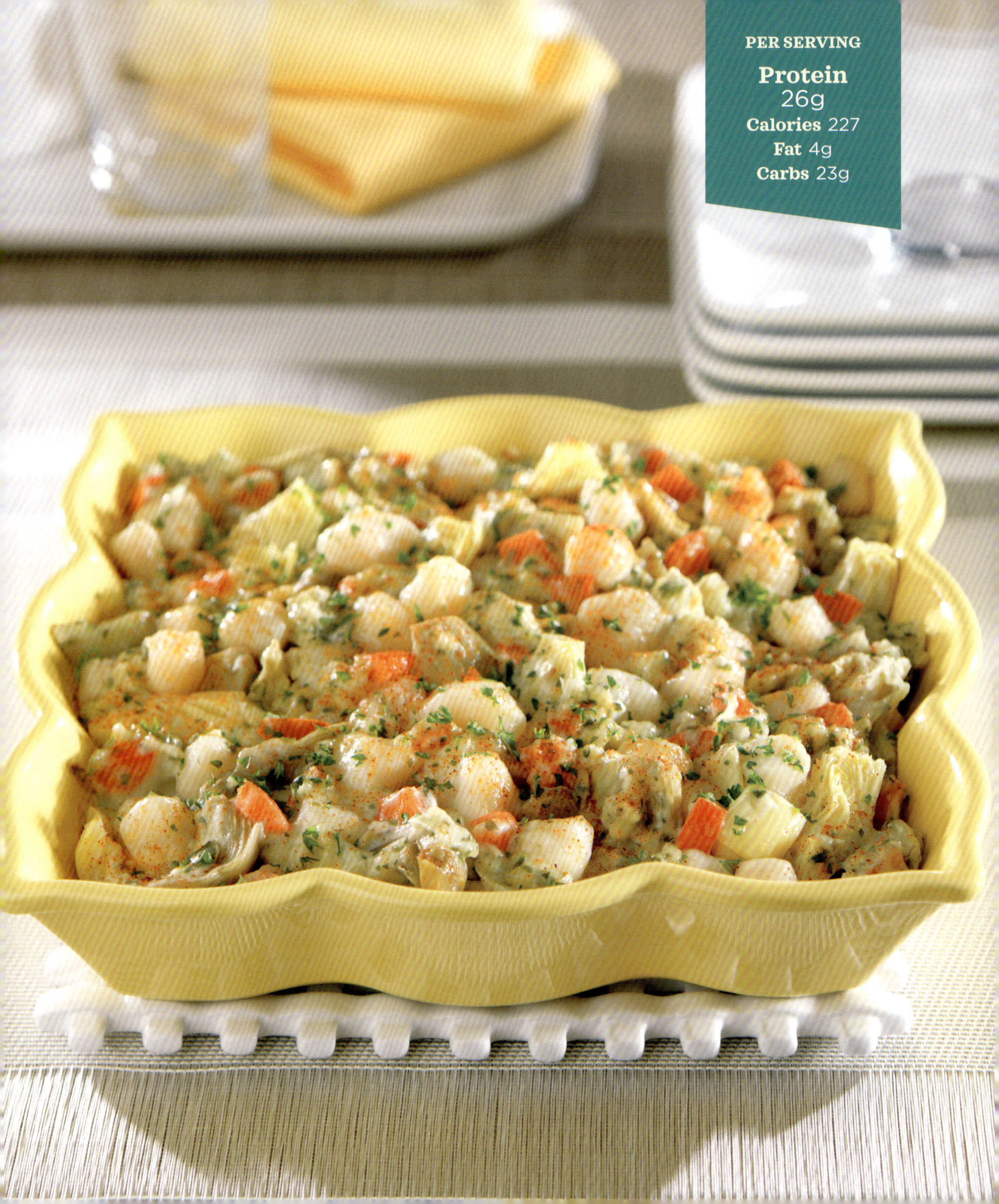
PER SERVING
Protein
26g
Calories 227
Fat 4g
Carbs 23g

Grilled Halibut with Cherry Tomato Relish

MAKES 4 SERVINGS

- 4 halibut fillets (about 6 ounces each)
- 3 tablespoons lemon juice, divided
- 2 teaspoons grated lemon peel, divided
- 2 cloves garlic, minced
- 2 teaspoons olive oil, divided
- ¼ teaspoon salt, divided
- ¼ teaspoon black pepper, divided
- 2 cups cherry tomatoes, quartered
- 2 tablespoons chopped fresh parsley

1. Place fish in large resealable food storage bag. Combine 2 tablespoons lemon juice, 1 teaspoon lemon peel, garlic, 1 teaspoon oil, ⅛ teaspoon salt and ⅛ teaspoon pepper in small bowl; mix well. Drizzle marinade over fish; seal bag and turn to coat. Marinate in refrigerator 1 hour.

2. Combine tomatoes, parsley, remaining 1 tablespoon lemon juice, 1 teaspoon lemon peel, 1 teaspoon oil, ⅛ teaspoon salt and ⅛ teaspoon pepper in medium bowl; mix well.

3. Spray grill grate with nonstick cooking spray. Prepare grill for direct cooking over medium-high heat. Remove fish from marinade; discard marinade.

4. Grill fish 3 to 5 minutes per side or until fish begins to flake when tested with fork. Serve with relish.

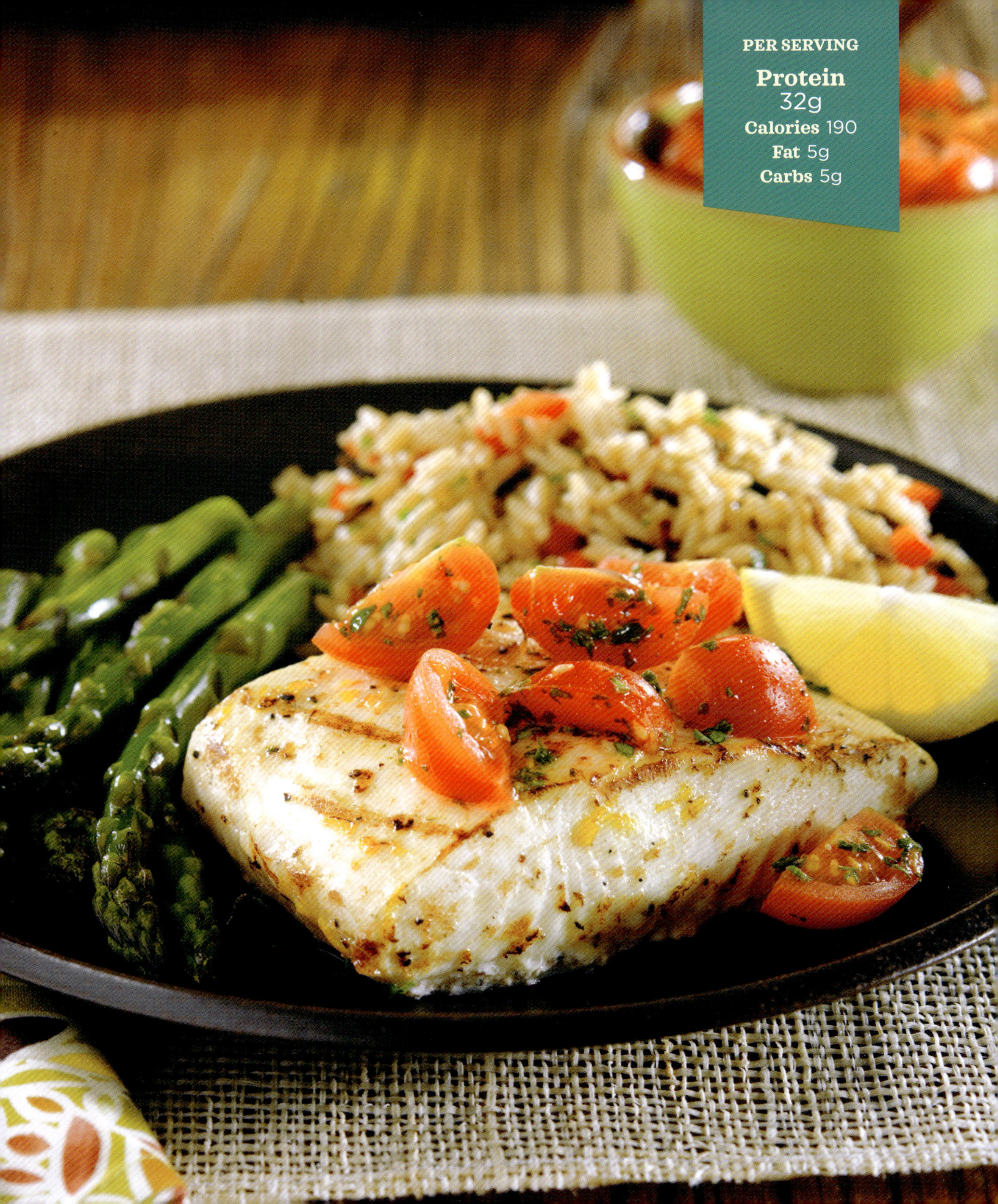
PER SERVING
Protein
32g
Calories 190
Fat 5g
Carbs 5g

Shrimp and Caper Vermicelli

MAKES 4 SERVINGS

- 1 medium tomato, seeded and chopped
- ¼ cup chopped fresh parsley
- 3 tablespoons capers, rinsed and drained
- 2 tablespoons dry white wine or reduced-sodium chicken broth
- 2 tablespoons lemon juice
- 1½ tablespoons olive oil
- 1 clove garlic, minced
- ½ teaspoon grated lemon peel
- ¼ teaspoon salt
- ⅛ to ¼ teaspoon red pepper flakes
- 6 ounces uncooked vermicelli, broken in thirds
- 10 ounces peeled fresh or thawed frozen raw medium shrimp
- 2 ounces reduced-fat feta cheese, crumbled (plain or basil and sun-dried tomato variety)

1. Combine tomato, parsley, capers, wine, lemon juice, oil, garlic, lemon peel, salt and red pepper flakes in large bowl; mix well.
2. Cook pasta in large saucepan according to package directions, omitting salt. After 6 minutes of cooking, add shrimp to saucepan. Return to a boil; cook 4 to 5 minutes or until shrimp is pink and opaque.
3. Drain pasta and shrimp; add to tomato mixture and toss to coat. Sprinkle with cheese; serve immediately.

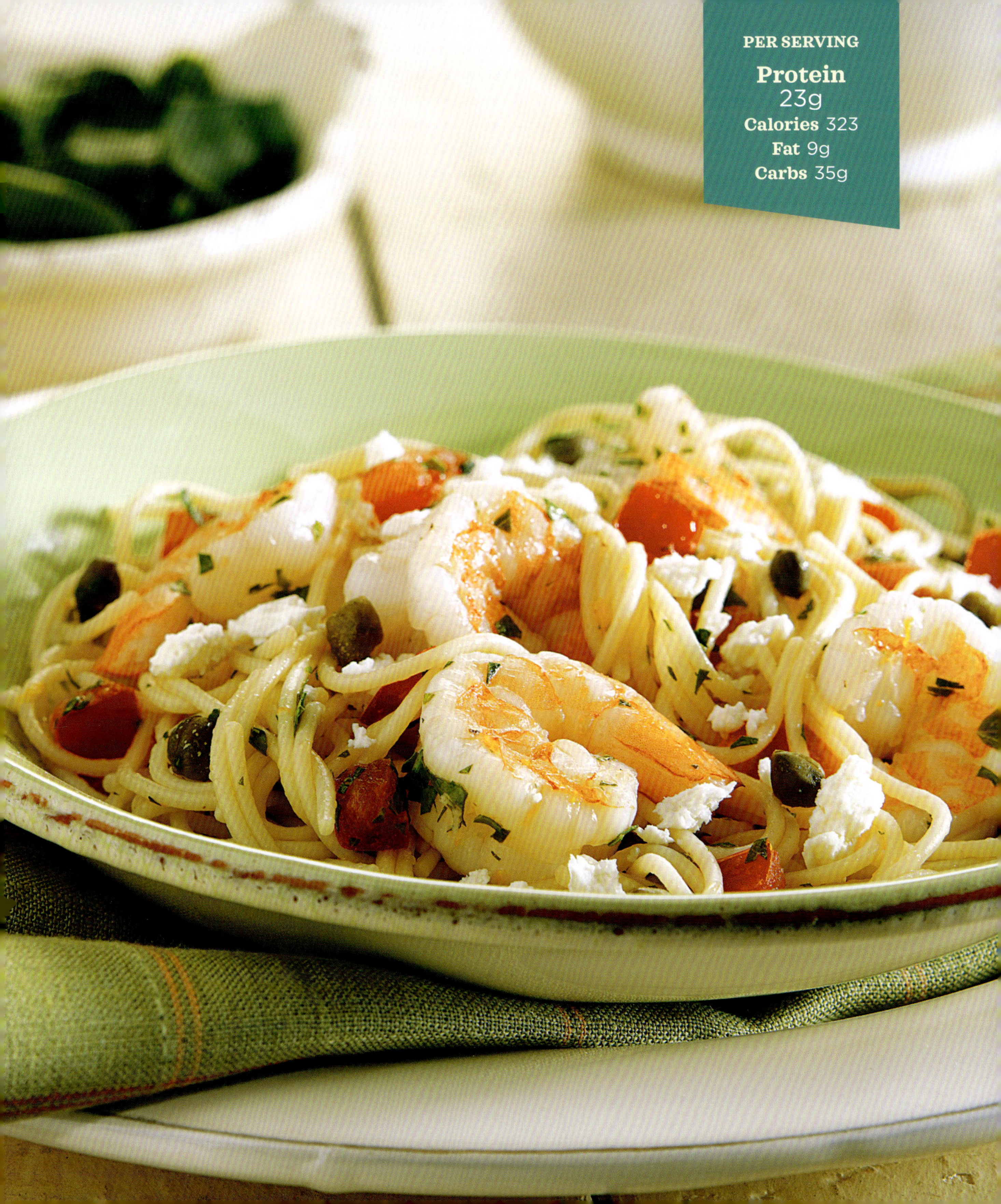
PER SERVING

Protein 23g

Calories 323

Fat 9g

Carbs 35g

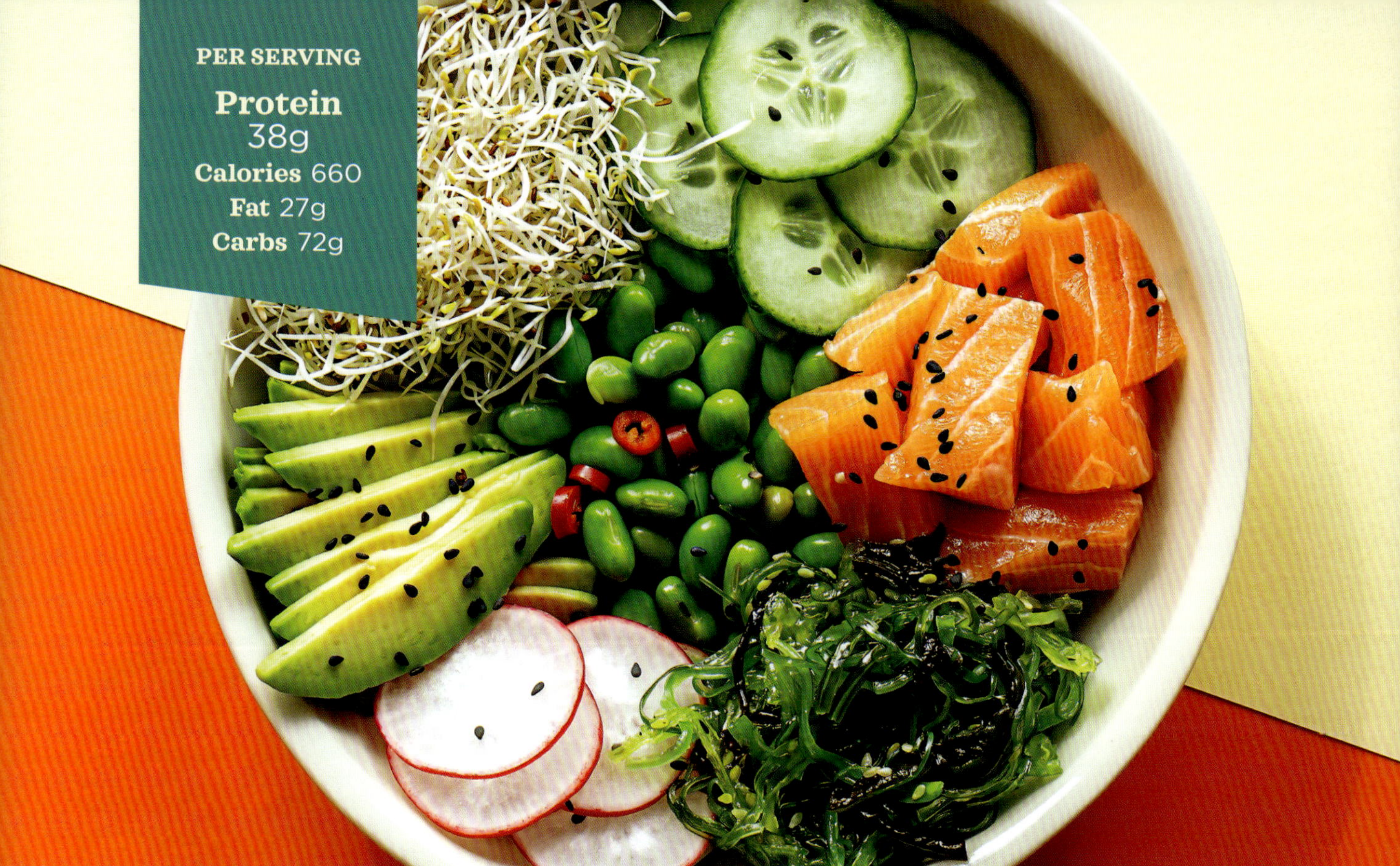

PER SERVING

Protein 38g
Calories 660
Fat 27g
Carbs 72g

Simple Sushi Poke Bowls

MAKES 2 SERVINGS

- 8 ounces sushi grade salmon
- 1½ cups cooked sushi rice or long grain rice
- 1 avocado, thinly sliced
- 1 mini cucumber, thinly sliced
- ⅔ cup thawed frozen shelled edamame
- ½ cup alfalfa sprouts
- ½ cup seaweed salad
- 2 radishes, thinly sliced
- 1 teaspoon black sesame seeds
- Prepared poke sauce

1. Cut salmon into ¾-inch cubes.
2. Divide rice between two bowls. Top with salmon, avocado, cucumber, edamame, alfalfa sprouts, seaweed salad and radishes.
3. Sprinkle with sesame seeds; serve with poke sauce.

Note

Seaweed salad and poke sauce can be found in Asian markets or the Asian section of large supermarkets.

PER SERVING
Protein
29g
Calories 243
Fat 12g
Carbs 3g

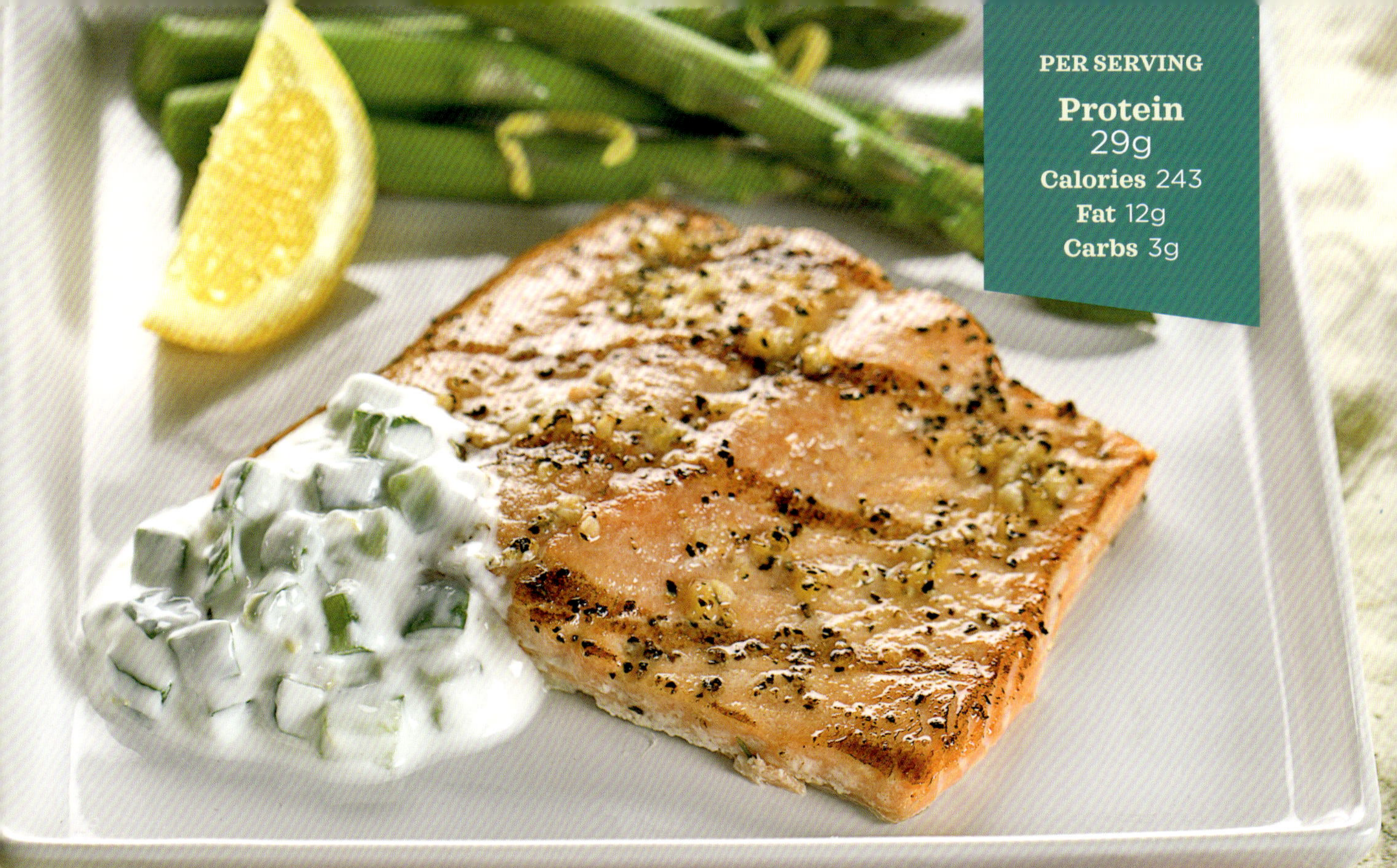

Lemon Garlic Salmon with Tzatziki Sauce

MAKES 4 SERVINGS

- ½ cup diced cucumber
- ¾ teaspoon salt, divided
- 1 cup plain nonfat Greek yogurt
- 2 tablespoons fresh lemon juice, divided
- 1 teaspoon grated lemon peel, divided
- 1 teaspoon minced garlic, divided
- ¼ teaspoon black pepper
- 4 skinless salmon fillets (4 ounces each)

1. Place cucumber in small colander set over small bowl; sprinkle with ¼ teaspoon salt. Set aside to drain 1 hour.

2. Combine yogurt, cucumber, 1 tablespoon lemon juice, ½ teaspoon lemon peel, ½ teaspoon garlic and ¼ teaspoon salt in small bowl; mix well. Cover and refrigerate until ready to use.

3. Combine remaining 1 tablespoon lemon juice, ½ teaspoon lemon peel, ½ teaspoon garlic, ¼ teaspoon salt and pepper in small bowl; mix well. Rub over fish.

4. Heat nonstick grill pan over medium-high heat. Cook fish 5 minutes per side or until fish begins to flake when tested with fork. Serve with sauce.

Pasta with Tuna, Green Beans and Tomatoes

MAKES 6 SERVINGS

- **8 ounces uncooked whole wheat penne, rigatoni or fusilli pasta**
- **1½ cups frozen cut green beans**
- **3 teaspoons olive oil, divided**
- **3 green onions, sliced**
- **1 clove garlic, minced**
- **1 can (about 14 ounces) diced Italian-style tomatoes, drained *or* 2 large tomatoes, chopped (about 2 cups)**
- **½ teaspoon salt**
- **½ teaspoon Italian seasoning**
- **¼ teaspoon black pepper**
- **1 can (12 ounces) solid albacore tuna packed in water, drained and flaked**

1. Cook pasta in large saucepan of boiling salted water according to package directions for al dente. Add green beans during last 7 minutes of cooking time (allow water to return to a boil before resuming timing). Drain and keep warm.

2. Meanwhile, heat 1 teaspoon oil in large skillet over medium heat. Add green onions and garlic; cook and stir 2 minutes. Add tomatoes, salt, Italian seasoning and pepper; cook and stir 4 to 5 minutes.

3. Add pasta and green bean mixture, tuna and remaining 2 teaspoons oil to skillet; stir gently to blend.

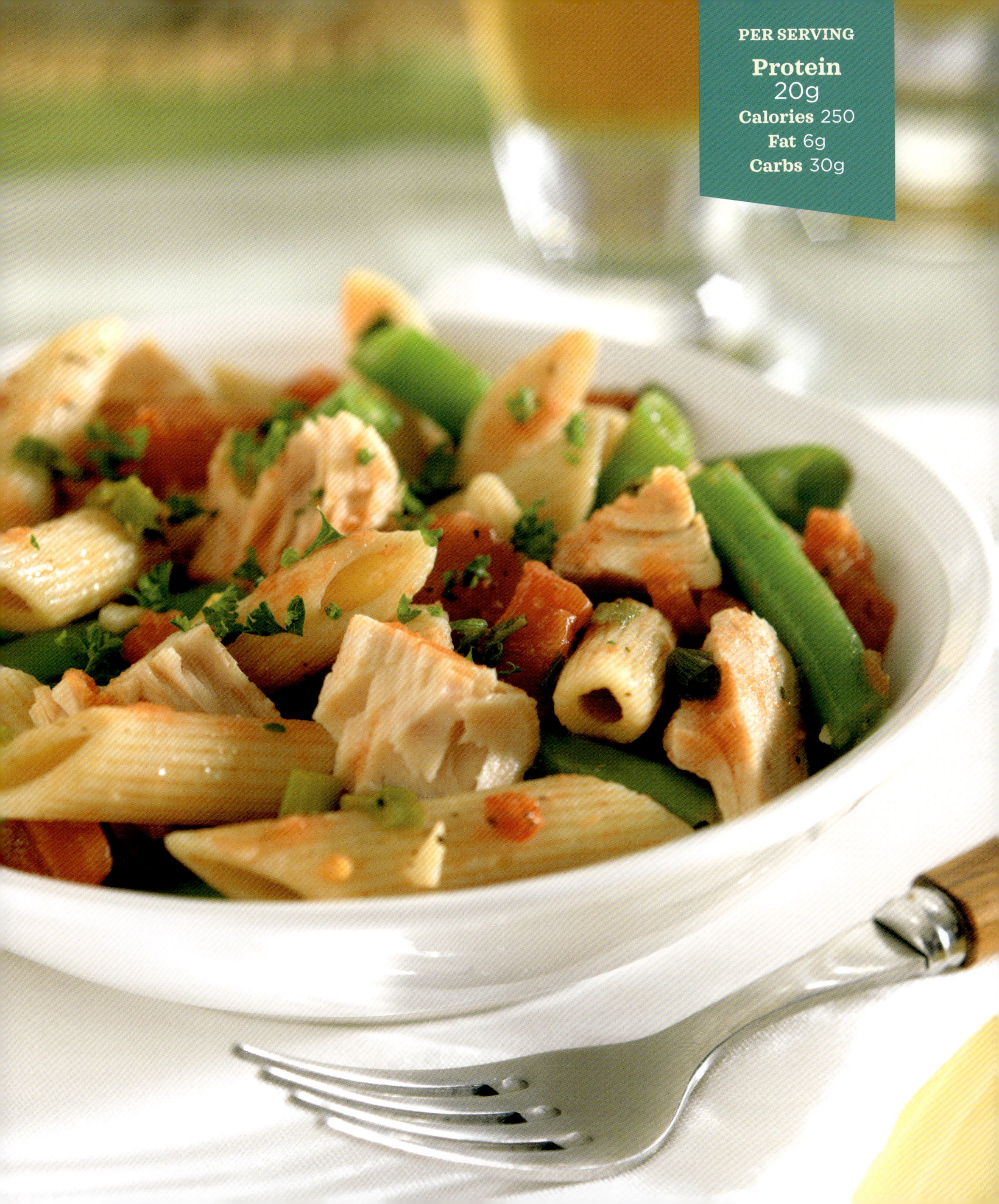
PER SERVING
Protein
20g
Calories 250
Fat 6g
Carbs 30g

Grilled Tilapia with Zesty Mustard Sauce

MAKES 4 SERVINGS

- 2 tablespoons light margarine or butter
- 1 teaspoon Dijon mustard
- ½ teaspoon grated lemon peel
- ½ teaspoon Worcestershire sauce
- ½ teaspoon salt, divided
- ¼ teaspoon black pepper
- 4 mild thin fish fillets, such as tilapia (about 4 ounces each)
- 1½ teaspoons paprika
- ½ medium lemon, quartered

1. Prepare grill for direct cooking over high heat. Spray grill basket with nonstick cooking spray.
2. Combine margarine, mustard, lemon peel, Worcestershire sauce, ¼ teaspoon salt and pepper in small bowl; mix well.
3. Rinse fish and pat dry. Sprinkle both sides of fish with paprika and remaining ¼ teaspoon salt. Place fish in prepared basket.
4. Grill fish, covered, 3 minutes; turn and grill, covered, 2 to 3 minutes or until fish begins to flake when tested with fork. Remove to plates.
5. Squeeze one lemon wedge over each fillet; spread margarine mixture evenly over fish.

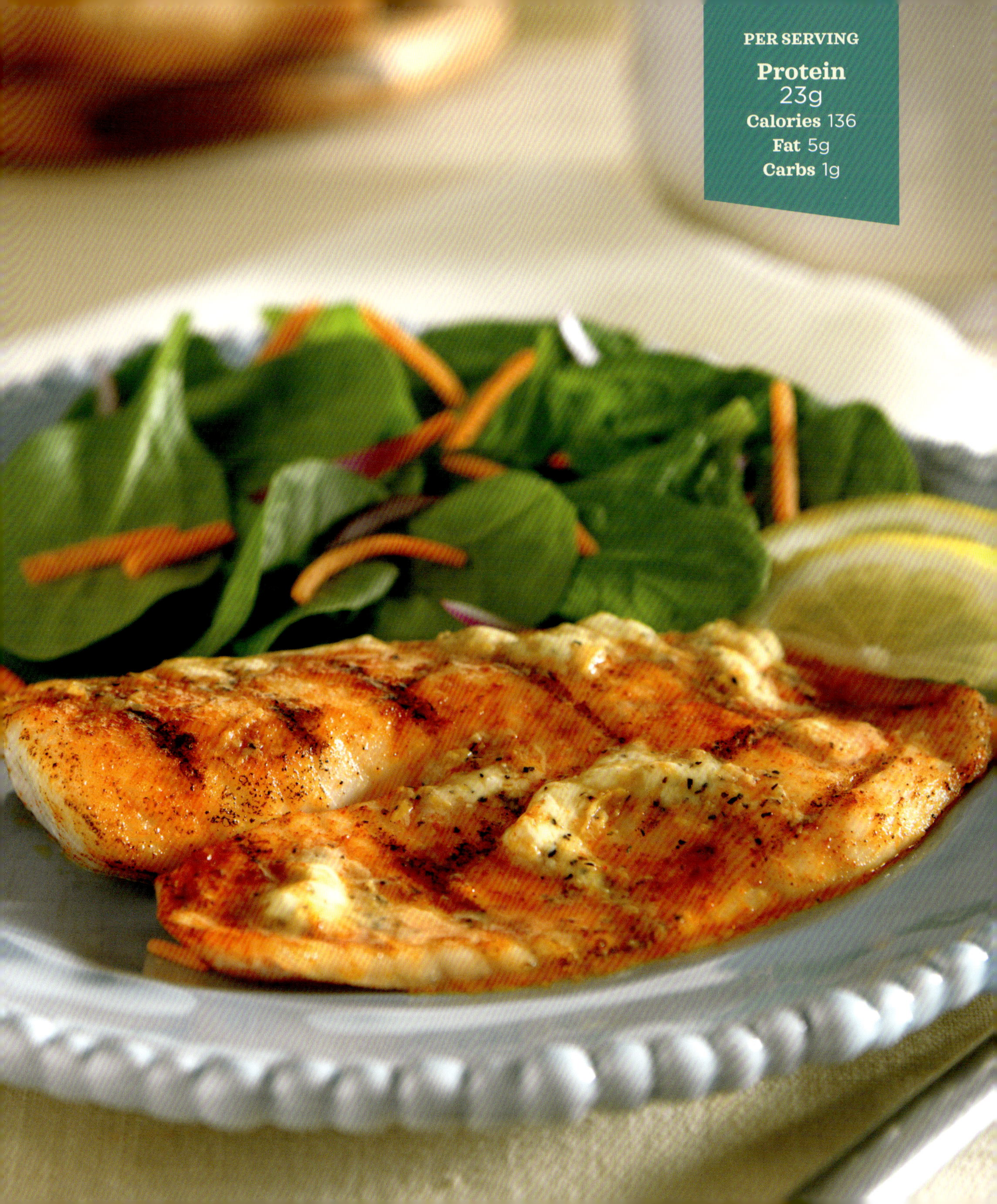
PER SERVING
Protein
23g
Calories 136
Fat 5g
Carbs 1g

Mediterranean Tuna Sandwiches

MAKES 4 SERVINGS

- 1 can (12 ounces) solid white tuna packed in water, drained
- ¼ cup finely chopped red onion
- ¼ cup fat-free or reduced-fat mayonnaise
- 3 tablespoons chopped black olives, drained
- 1 tablespoon plus 1 teaspoon lemon juice
- 1 tablespoon olive oil
- 1 tablespoon chopped fresh mint (optional)
- ¼ teaspoon black pepper
- ⅛ teaspoon garlic powder (optional)
- 8 slices whole wheat bread
- 8 leaves romaine lettuce
- 8 thin slices tomato

1 Combine tuna, onion, mayonnaise, olives, lemon juice, oil, mint, if desired, pepper and garlic powder, if desired, in large bowl; stir gently to blend.

2 Place lettuce and tomato on each of four bread slices; top with ⅔ cup tuna mixture and remaining bread slices. Cut sandwiches in half.

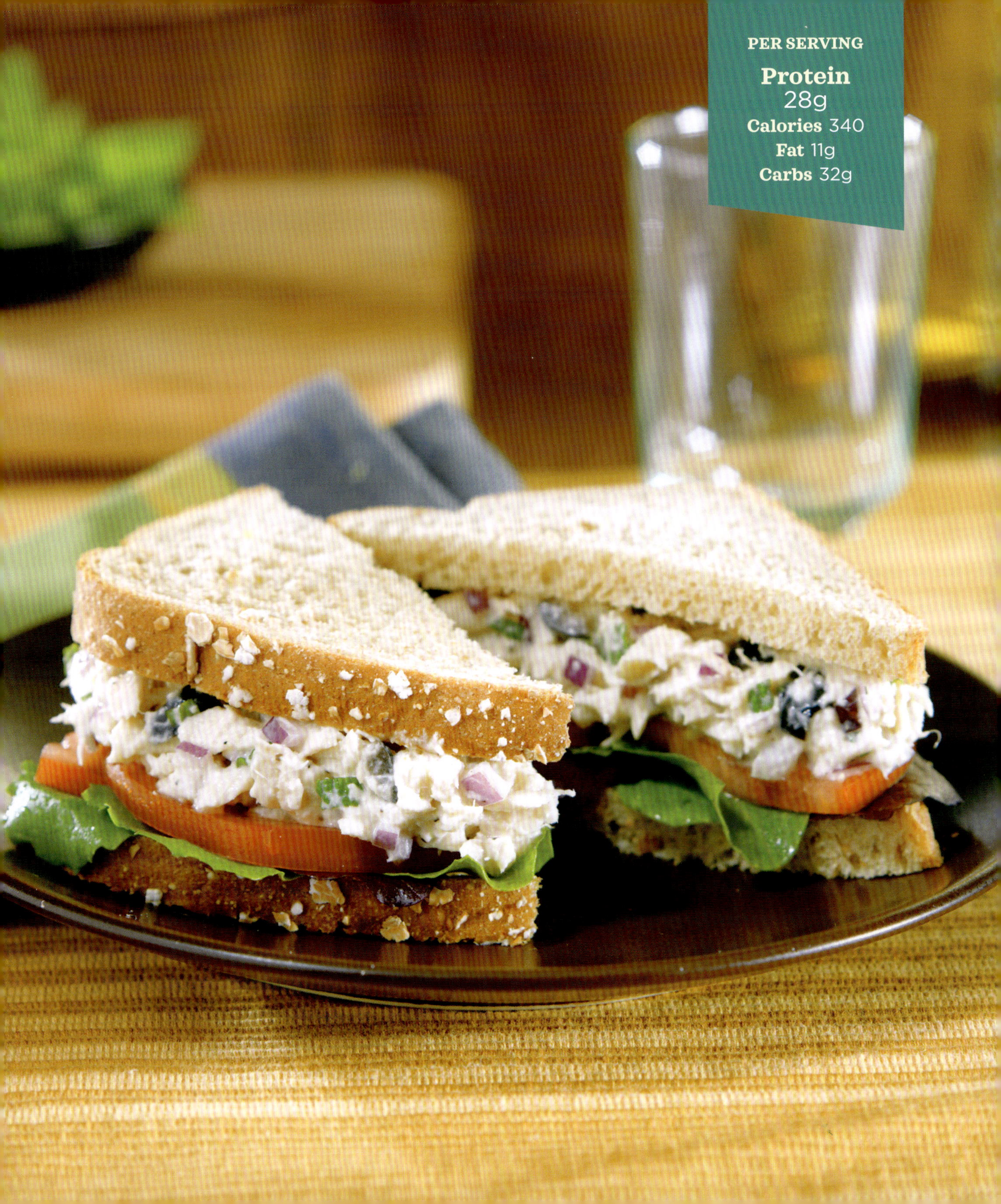
PER SERVING
Protein
28g
Calories 340
Fat 11g
Carbs 32g

PER SERVING
Protein
24g
Calories 144
Fat 2g
Carbs 7g

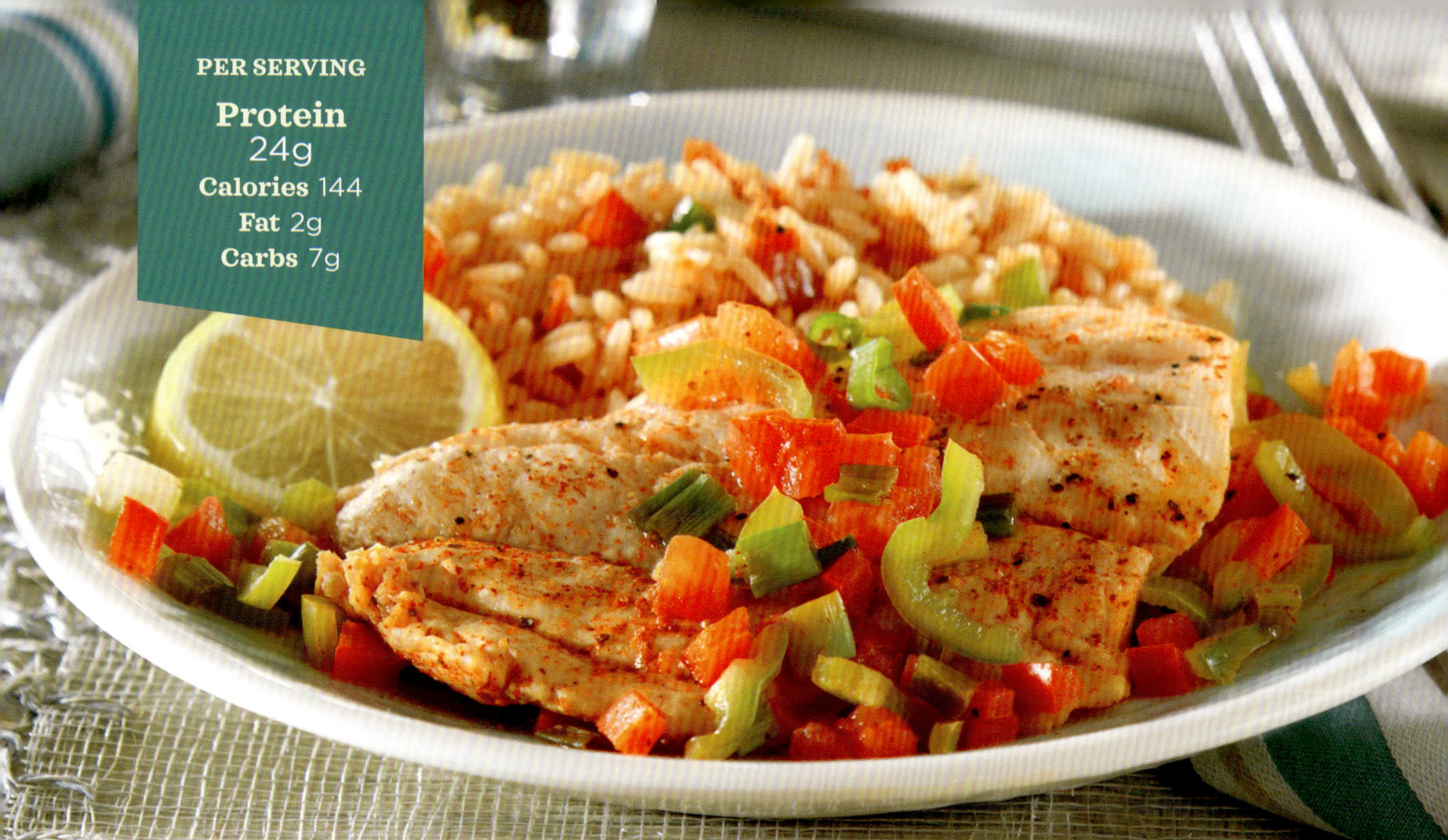

Red Snapper Vera Cruz

MAKES 4 SERVINGS

- 4 red snapper fillets (about 4 ounces each)
- ¼ cup lime juice
- 1 tablespoon lemon juice
- 1 teaspoon chili powder
- 4 green onions, cut into ½-inch lengths
- 1 tomato, coarsely chopped
- ½ cup chopped Anaheim or green bell pepper
- ½ cup chopped red bell pepper
- Black pepper

1. Place fish in shallow 9- to 10-inch round microwavable dish. Combine lime juice, lemon juice and chili powder in small bowl; mix well. Pour over fish; marinate 10 minutes, turning once or twice.

2. Sprinkle green onions, tomato, Anaheim pepper and bell pepper over fish; season with black pepper. Cover loosely with vented plastic wrap.

3. Microwave on HIGH 5 to 6 minutes or just until fish begins to flake with tested with fork, turning dish every 2 minutes. Let stand, covered, 4 minutes before serving.

PER SERVING
Protein
28g
Calories 172
Fat 5g
Carbs 3g

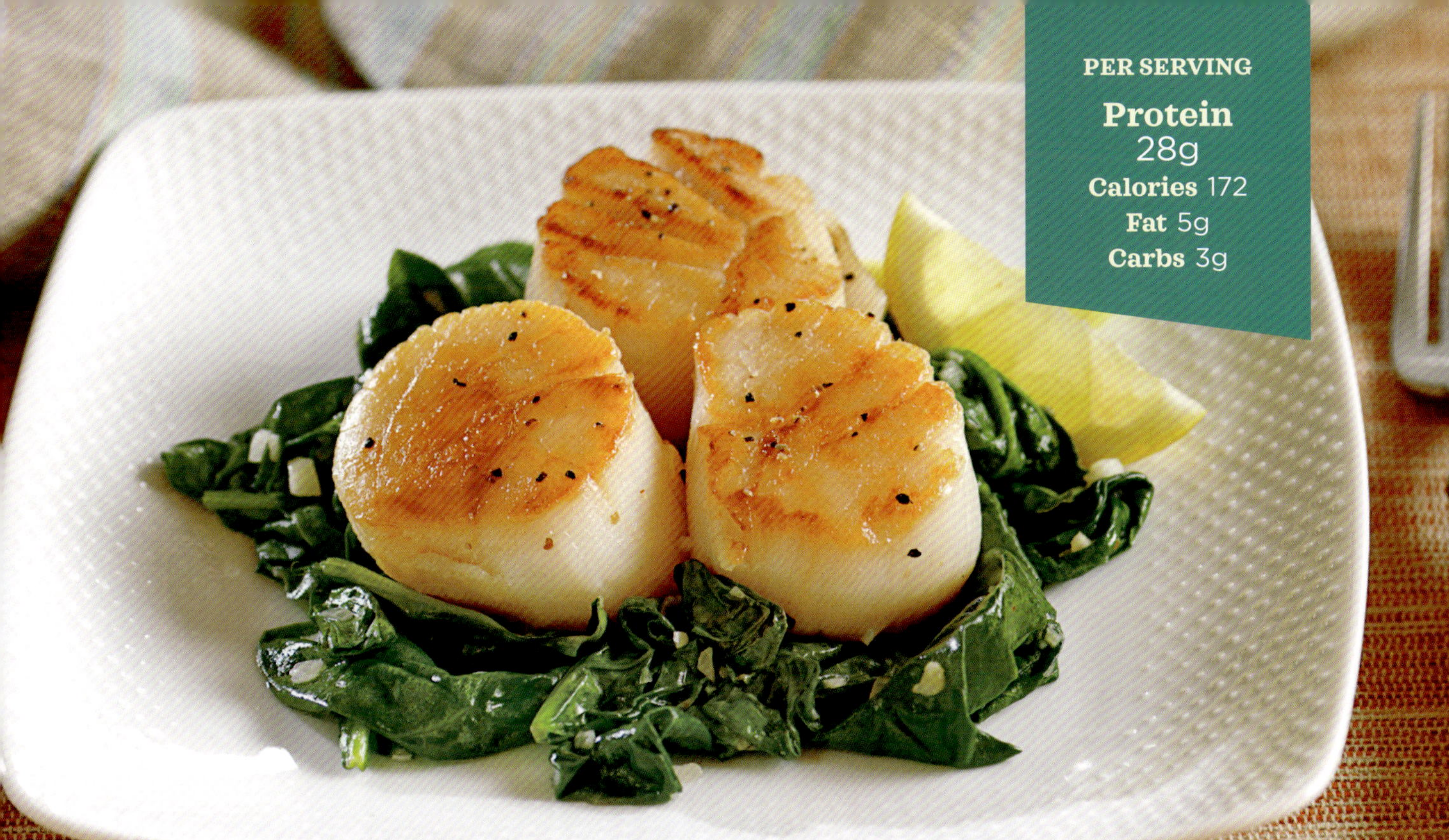

Seared Scallops over Garlic-Lemon Spinach

MAKES 4 SERVINGS

1 tablespoon olive oil
1 pound sea scallops (about 12)
¼ teaspoon salt
⅛ teaspoon black pepper
2 cloves garlic, minced
1 shallot, minced
1 package (about 5 ounces) baby spinach
1 tablespoon lemon juice
Lemon wedges (optional)

1 Heat oil in large nonstick skillet over medium-high heat. Pat scallops dry with paper towel. Add scallops to skillet; sprinkle with salt and pepper. Cook 2 to 3 minutes per side or until golden brown. Remove to plate; tent with foil to keep warm.

2 Add garlic and shallot to skillet; cook and stir 45 seconds or until fragrant. Add spinach; cook 2 minutes or just until spinach begins to wilt, stirring occasionally. Remove from heat; stir in lemon juice.

3 Serve scallops over spinach. Serve with lemon wedges, if desired.

Impossibly Easy Salmon Pie

MAKES 8 SERVINGS

- **1 can (7½ ounces) red salmon, drained and deboned**
- **½ cup grated Parmesan cheese**
- **¼ cup sliced green onions**
- **1 jar (2 ounces) chopped pimientos, drained**
- **½ cup low-fat (1%) cottage cheese**
- **1 tablespoon lemon juice**
- **1½ cups low-fat (1%) milk**
- **¾ cup reduced-fat biscuit baking mix**
- **2 eggs**
- **2 egg whites *or* ¼ cup liquid egg substitute**
- **¼ teaspoon salt**
- **¼ teaspoon dried dill weed**
- **¼ teaspoon paprika (optional)**

1 Preheat oven to 375°F. Spray 9-inch pie plate with nonstick cooking spray.

2 Combine salmon, Parmesan, green onions and pimientos in prepared pie plate; mix well.

3 Combine cottage cheese and lemon juice in blender or food processor; blend until smooth. Add milk, baking mix, eggs, egg whites, salt and dill weed; blend 15 seconds. Pour over salmon mixture in pie plate; sprinkle with paprika, if desired.

4 Bake 35 to 40 minutes or until top is golden brown and knife inserted into center comes out clean. Let stand 5 minutes before serving.

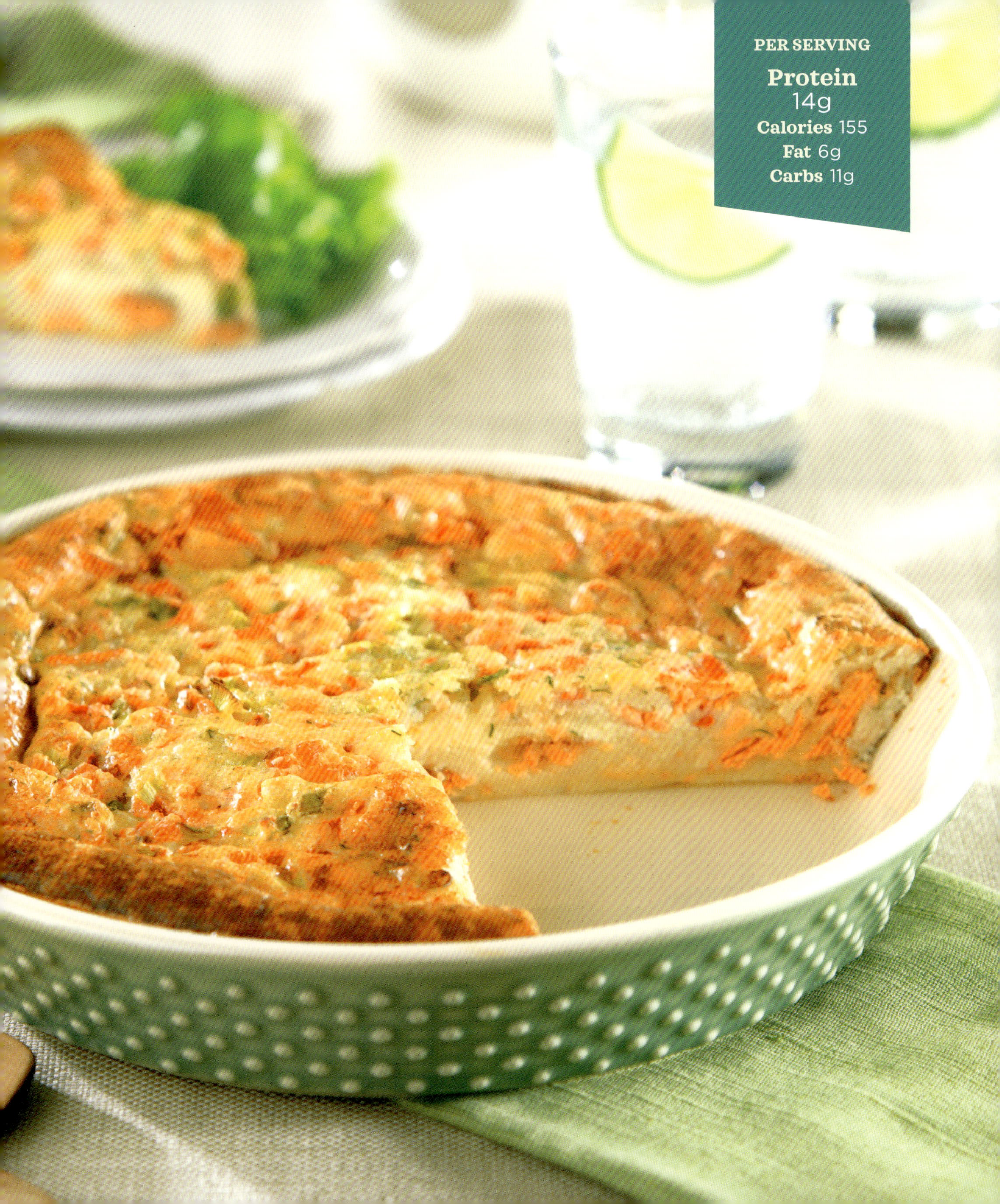
PER SERVING
Protein
14g
Calories 155
Fat 6g
Carbs 11g

Shrimp and Tomato Stir-Fry

MAKES 4 SERVINGS

- 1 cup cherry tomatoes, halved
- 20 Kalamata olives, pitted and coarsely chopped
- ¼ cup chopped fresh basil
- ¼ teaspoon plus ⅛ teaspoon salt, divided
- ¼ teaspoon black pepper
- 1 pound medium raw shrimp, peeled and deveined
- 1 clove garlic, minced
- ⅛ teaspoon red pepper flakes
- 1 medium zucchini, quartered lengthwise, then cut crosswise into 2-inch pieces
- 1 medium onion, cut into 8 wedges

1. Combine tomatoes, olives, basil, ⅛ teaspoon salt and pepper in small bowl; mix well.

2. Spray large nonstick skillet with nonstick cooking spray; heat over medium heat. Add shrimp, garlic and pepper flakes; cook and stir 3 minutes or until shrimp are opaque. Remove to medium bowl.

3. Spray same skillet with cooking spray; heat over medium-high heat. Add zucchini, onion and remaining ¼ teaspoon salt; cook and stir 5 minutes or until edges of vegetables begin to brown.

4. Add tomato mixture and shrimp to skillet; cook and stir 1 minute or until heated through.

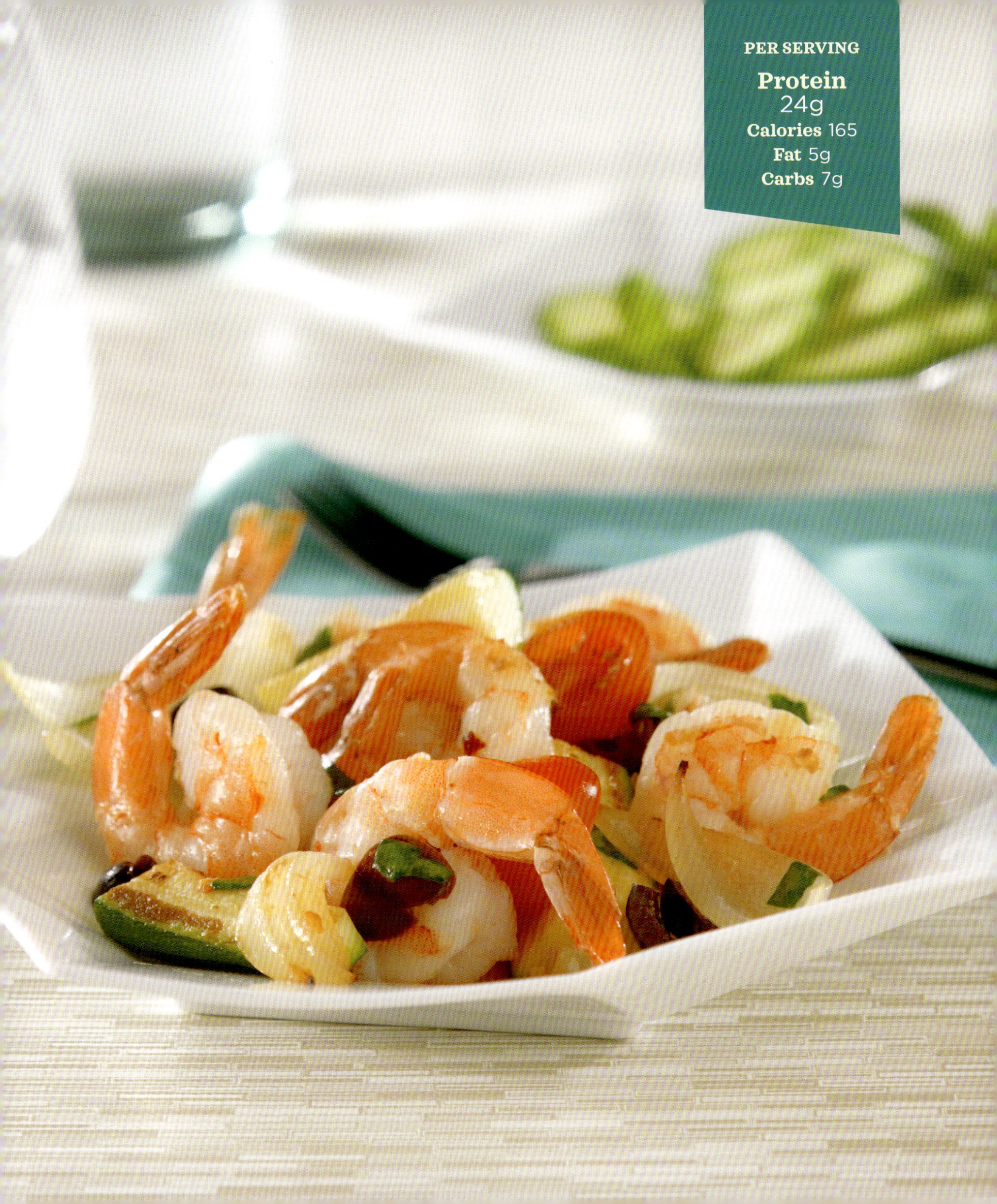
PER SERVING
Protein
24g
Calories 165
Fat 5g
Carbs 7g

Baked Fish with Thai Pesto

MAKES 6 SERVINGS

- 1½ cups lightly packed fresh basil leaves
- 1 cup lightly packed fresh cilantro leaves
- 4 green onions, thinly sliced, plus additional for garnish
- ¼ cup lightly packed fresh mint leaves
- ¼ cup unsalted roasted peanuts
- 2 tablespoons chopped fresh ginger
- 2 tablespoons sweetened shredded coconut
- 1 to 2 jalapeño peppers, coarsely chopped
- Grated peel and juice of 1 lemon
- 3 cloves garlic, minced
- ½ teaspoon sugar
- ½ cup peanut oil
- 2 pounds boneless fish fillets (such as salmon, halibut, cod or orange roughy)

1. Combine basil, cilantro, 4 green onions, mint, peanuts, ginger, coconut, jalapeños, lemon peel, lemon juice, garlic and sugar in blender or food processor; blend until finely chopped. With motor running, slowly pour in oil; blend until almost smooth.
2. Preheat oven to 375°F. Spray baking sheet with nonstick cooking spray or line with parchment paper.
3. Rinse fish and pat dry with paper towel. Place on prepared baking sheet; spread solid thin layer of pesto over each fillet.
4. Bake fish 10 minutes or until fish is opaque in center and begins to flake when tested with fork. Garnish as desired.

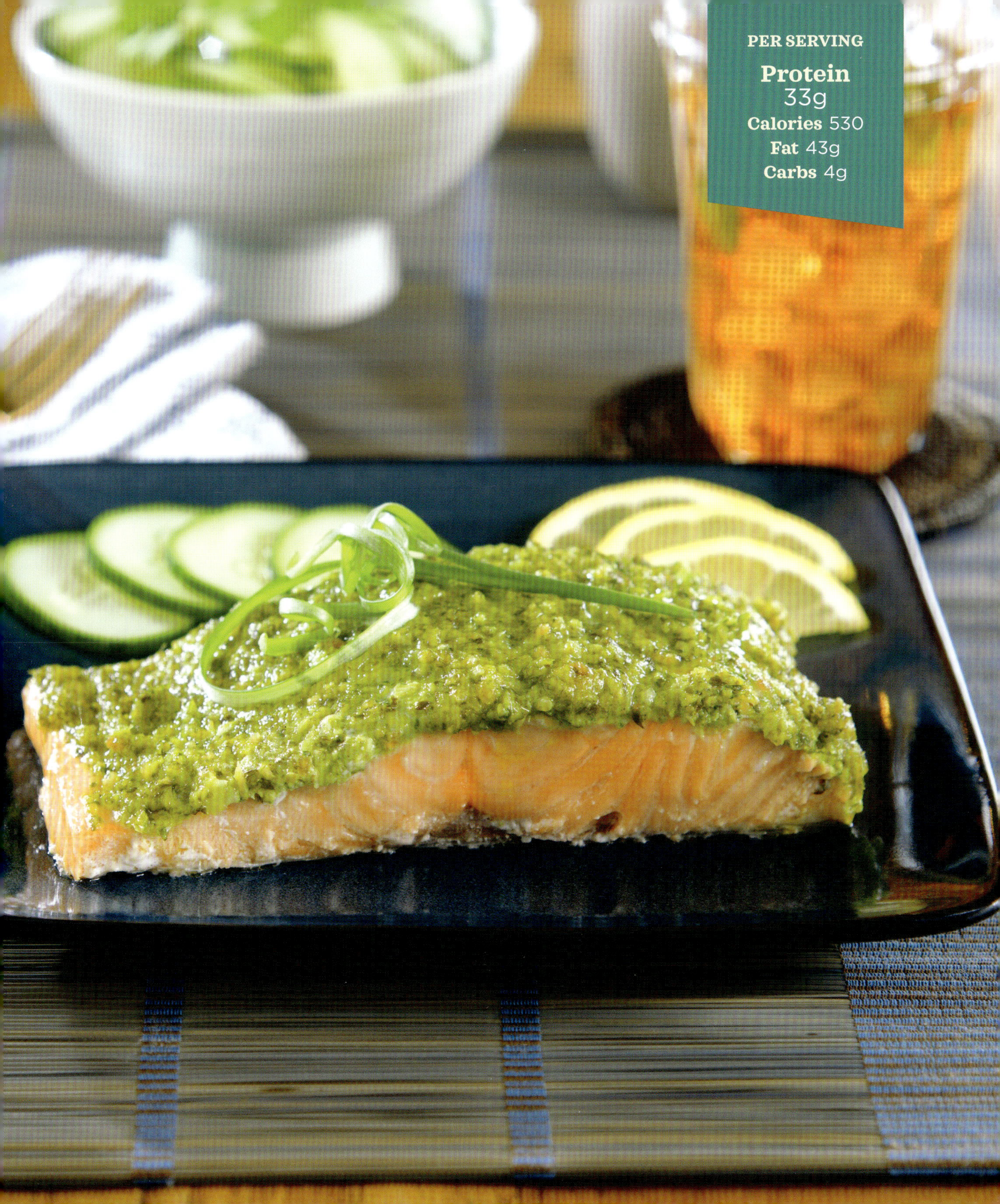
PER SERVING
Protein
33g
Calories 530
Fat 43g
Carbs 4g

PER SERVING
Protein
26g
Calories 193
Fat 9g
Carbs 3g

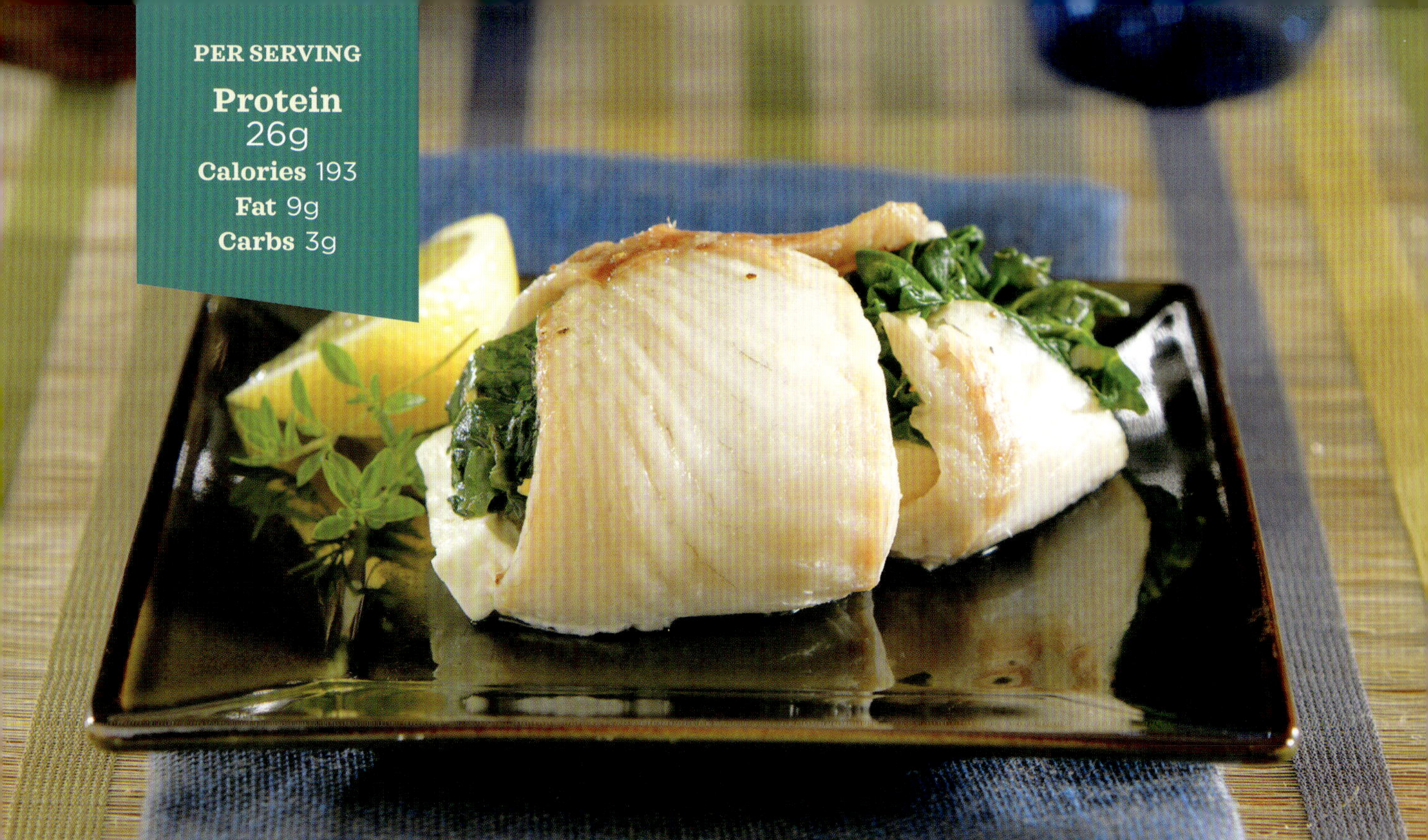

Tilapia with Spinach and Feta

MAKES 2 SERVINGS

- 1 teaspoon olive oil
- 1 clove garlic, minced
- 4 cups baby spinach
- 2 skinless tilapia fillets or other mild white fish (4 ounces each)
- ¼ teaspoon black pepper
- 2 ounces reduced-fat feta cheese, cut into 2 (3-inch) pieces

1 Preheat oven to 350°F. Spray baking sheet with nonstick cooking spray.

2 Heat oil in medium skillet over medium-low heat. Add garlic; cook and stir 30 seconds. Add spinach; cook 2 minutes or just until wilted, stirring occasionally.

3 Place fish on prepared baking sheet; sprinkle with pepper. Place one piece of cheese on each fillet; top with spinach mixture. Fold one end of each fillet up and over filling; secure with toothpick. Repeat with opposite end of each fillet.

4 Bake fish 20 minutes or until fish begins to flake when tested with fork.

PER SERVING
Protein
16g
Calories 205
Fat 10g
Carbs 13g

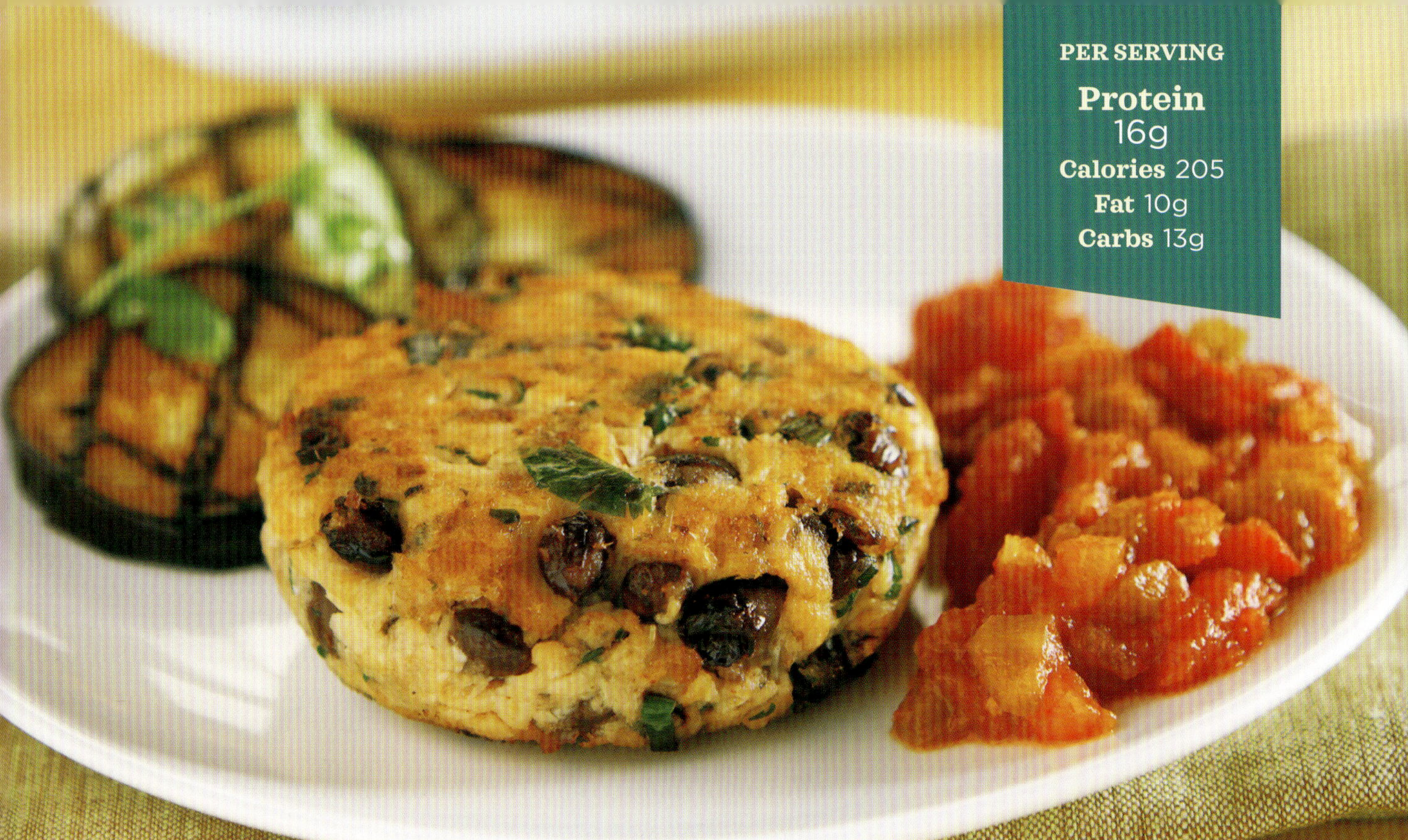

Salmon Black Bean Patties

MAKES 3 PATTIES

- 1 can (7½ ounces) pink salmon, drained
- ½ cup no-salt-added black beans, rinsed and drained
- ¼ cup plain dry bread crumbs
- ¼ cup sliced green onions
- 1 egg white
- 1 tablespoon chopped fresh cilantro
- 1 tablespoon lime juice
- ⅛ teaspoon black pepper
- Pinch ground red pepper or seafood seasoning mix
- 1 tablespoon canola oil

1. Place salmon in medium bowl; shred with fork.
2. Add beans, bread crumbs, green onions, egg white, cilantro, lime juice, black pepper and red pepper; mix well.
3. Shape mixture into three patties about 1¼ inches thick. Refrigerate 30 minutes or until ready to cook.
4. Heat oil in large skillet over medium heat. Add patties; cook 2 to 3 minutes per side or until golden brown.

Grilled Scallops and Vegetables with Cilantro Sauce

MAKES 4 SERVINGS

- **1 teaspoon hot chili oil**
- **1 teaspoon dark sesame oil**
- **1 green onion, chopped**
- **1 tablespoon finely chopped fresh ginger**
- **1 cup reduced-sodium chicken broth**
- **1 cup chopped fresh cilantro**
- **1 pound raw or thawed frozen sea scallops**
- **2 medium zucchini, cut into ½-inch slices**
- **2 medium yellow squash, cut into ½-inch slices**
- **1 medium yellow onion, cut into wedges**
- **8 large mushrooms**

1. Spray grill grate with nonstick cooking spray. Prepare grill for direct cooking over medium-high heat.
2. Heat chili oil and sesame oil in small saucepan over medium-low heat. Add green onion; cook and stir about 15 seconds or just until fragrant. Add ginger; cook and stir 1 minute. Stir in broth; bring to a boil. Cook until liquid is reduced by half; set aside to cool slightly.
3. Pour broth mixture into blender or food processor; add cilantro and blend until smooth. (Or add cilantro to saucepan and use immersion blender to blend mixture until smooth.)
4. Thread scallops and vegetables onto four 12-inch skewers.*
5. Grill skewers about 8 minutes per side or until scallops are opaque. Serve immediately with cilantro sauce.

**If using wooden skewers, soak in cold water 20 to 30 minutes to prevent burning.*

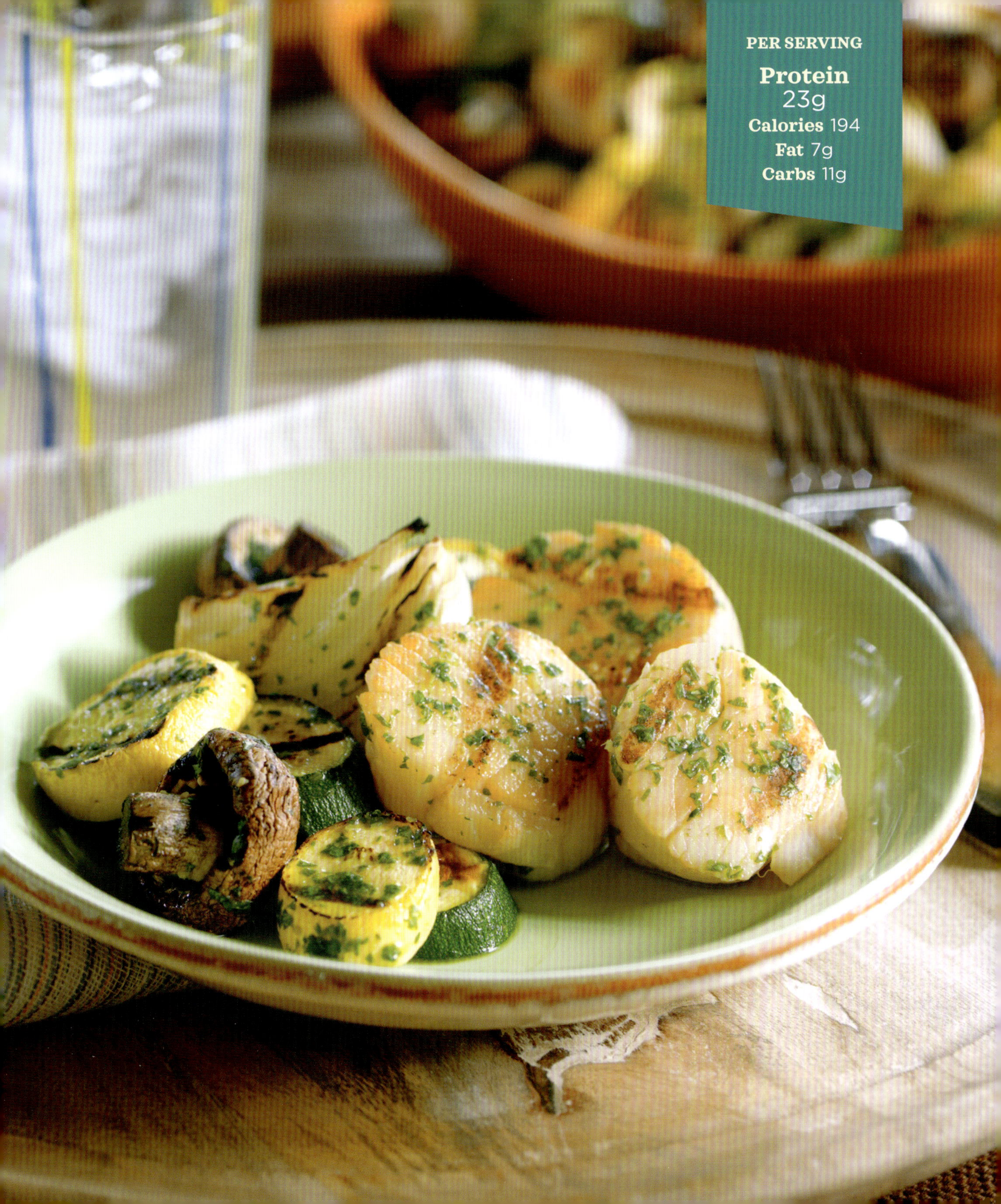
PER SERVING
Protein
23g
Calories 194
Fat 7g
Carbs 11g

Szechuan Tuna Steaks

MAKES 4 SERVINGS

- **4 tuna steaks (6 ounces each, about 1 inch thick)**
- **¼ cup dry sherry or sake**
- **¼ cup soy sauce**
- **1 tablespoon dark sesame oil**
- **1 teaspoon hot chili oil *or* ¼ teaspoon red pepper flakes**
- **1 clove garlic, minced**
- **2 tablespoons chopped fresh cilantro (optional)**

1. Place fish in single layer in large shallow dish. Combine sherry, soy sauce, sesame oil, hot chili oil and garlic in small bowl; mix well.
2. Reserve ¼ cup soy sauce mixture in another small bowl for serving. Pour remaining mixture over fish; cover and marinate in refrigerator 40 minutes, turning once.
3. Spray grill grate with nonstick cooking spray. Prepare grill for direct cooking over medium-high heat. Drain fish; discard marinade.
4. Grill fish about 3 minutes per side or until fish is seared but still feels somewhat soft in center.* Remove to cutting board; let rest 5 minutes.
5. Cut fish into thin slices; drizzle with reserved soy sauce mixture. Garnish with cilantro.

**Tuna becomes dry and tough if overcooked. Cook to medium doneness for best results.*

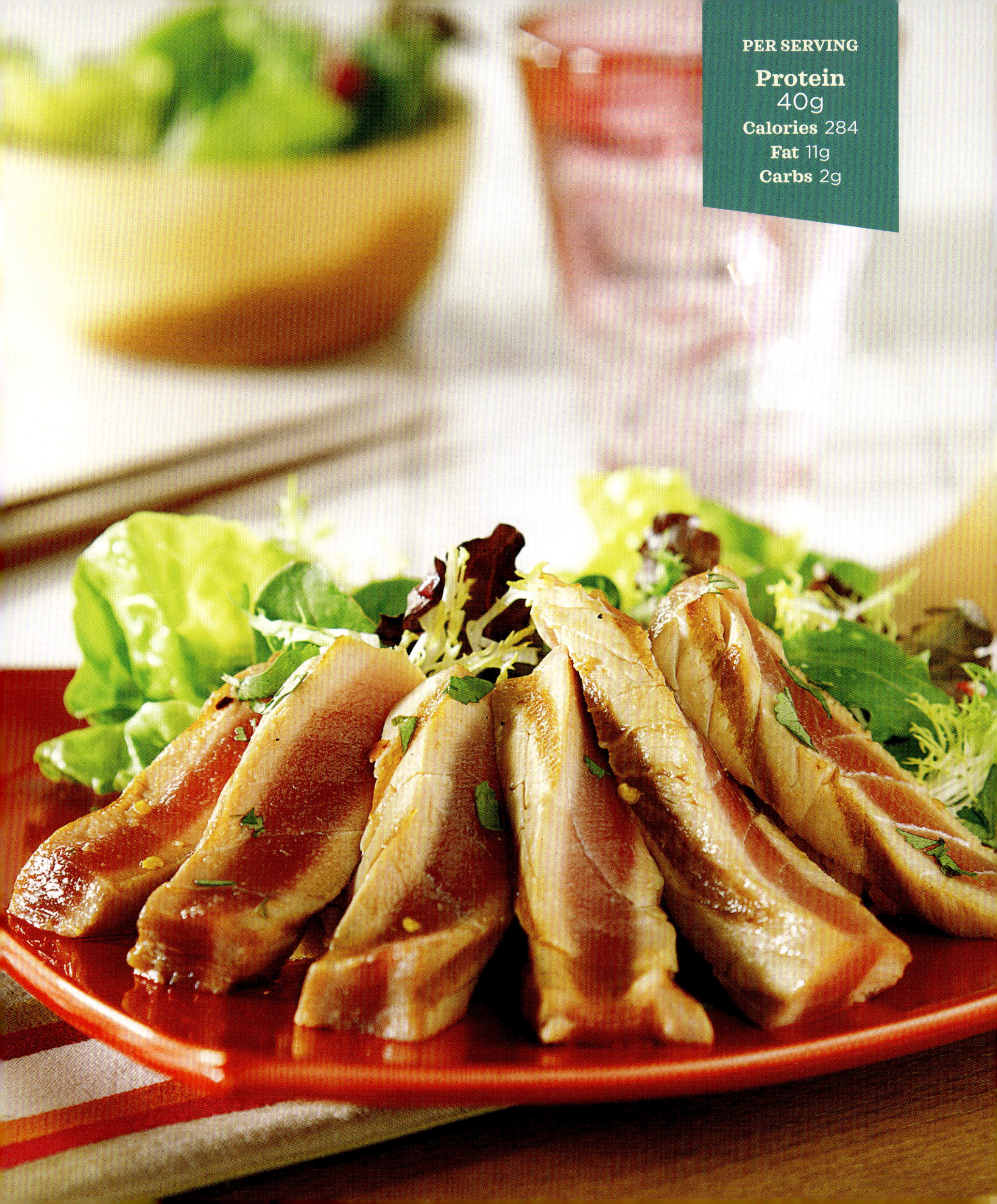
PER SERVING
Protein
40g
Calories 284
Fat 11g
Carbs 2g

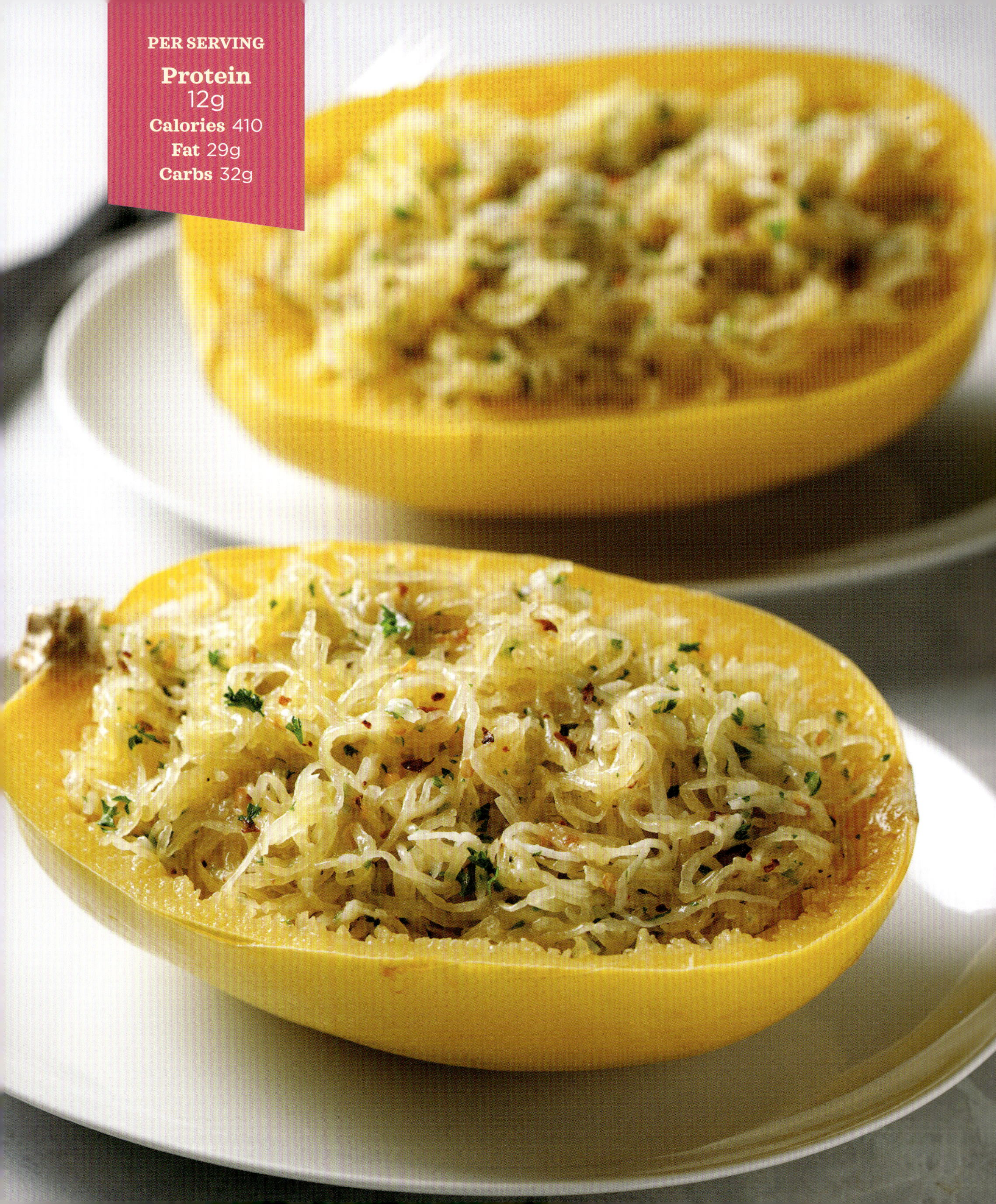
PER SERVING
Protein
12g
Calories 410
Fat 29g
Carbs 32g

MEATLESS

Garlic Parmesan Spaghetti Squash

MAKES 2 SERVINGS

- **3 tablespoons olive oil, divided**
- **1 medium spaghetti squash (2 to 2½ pounds)**
- **¼ teaspoon plus ⅛ teaspoon salt, divided**
- **1 clove garlic, minced**
- **¼ teaspoon red pepper flakes**
- **⅛ teaspoon black pepper**
- **½ cup shredded Parmesan cheese**
- **⅓ cup chopped fresh parsley**

1. Preheat oven to 400°F. Brush baking sheet with 1 teaspoon oil. Cut squash in half; remove and discard seeds. Brush each cut side with 1 teaspoon oil and sprinkle each half with ⅛ teaspoon salt. Place squash cut sides down on prepared baking sheet.
2. Bake 30 to 40 minutes or until squash is fork-tender.
3. Remove squash to plate; let stand until cool enough to handle. Use fork to shred squash into long strands, reserving shells for serving, if desired.
4. Heat remaining 2 tablespoons oil in large nonstick skillet over medium-high heat. Add garlic, red pepper flakes, black pepper and remaining ⅛ teaspoon salt; cook and stir 2 to 3 minutes or until garlic begins to turn golden. Remove from heat. Add squash, cheese and parsley to skillet; stir gently just until blended. Serve immediately.

Lentil Ragù

MAKES 8 SERVINGS

- 2 tablespoons olive oil
- 1 onion, chopped
- 1 carrot, chopped
- 1 stalk celery, chopped
- 2 cloves garlic, minced
- 1 teaspoon salt
- ½ teaspoon dried oregano
- Pinch red pepper flakes
- 3 tablespoons tomato paste
- ¼ cup dry white wine
- 1 can (28 ounces) crushed tomatoes
- 1 can (about 14 ounces) diced tomatoes
- 1½ cups water
- 1 cup dried lentils, rinsed and sorted
- 1 portobello mushroom, gills removed, finely chopped
- 1 package (16 ounces) uncooked whole wheat rotini

1. Heat oil in large saucepan over medium heat. Add onion, carrot and celery; cook and stir 10 minutes or until onion is lightly browned and carrot is softened.

2. Stir in garlic, salt, oregano and red pepper flakes. Add tomato paste; cook and stir 1 minute. Add wine; cook and stir until wine is absorbed.

3. Stir in crushed tomatoes, diced tomatoes, water, lentils and mushroom; bring to a simmer. Reduce heat to medium-low; partially cover and simmer 20 minutes. Uncover; simmer 20 minutes or until lentils are tender.

4. Cook pasta according to package directions for al dente. Drain and serve with lentil ragù.

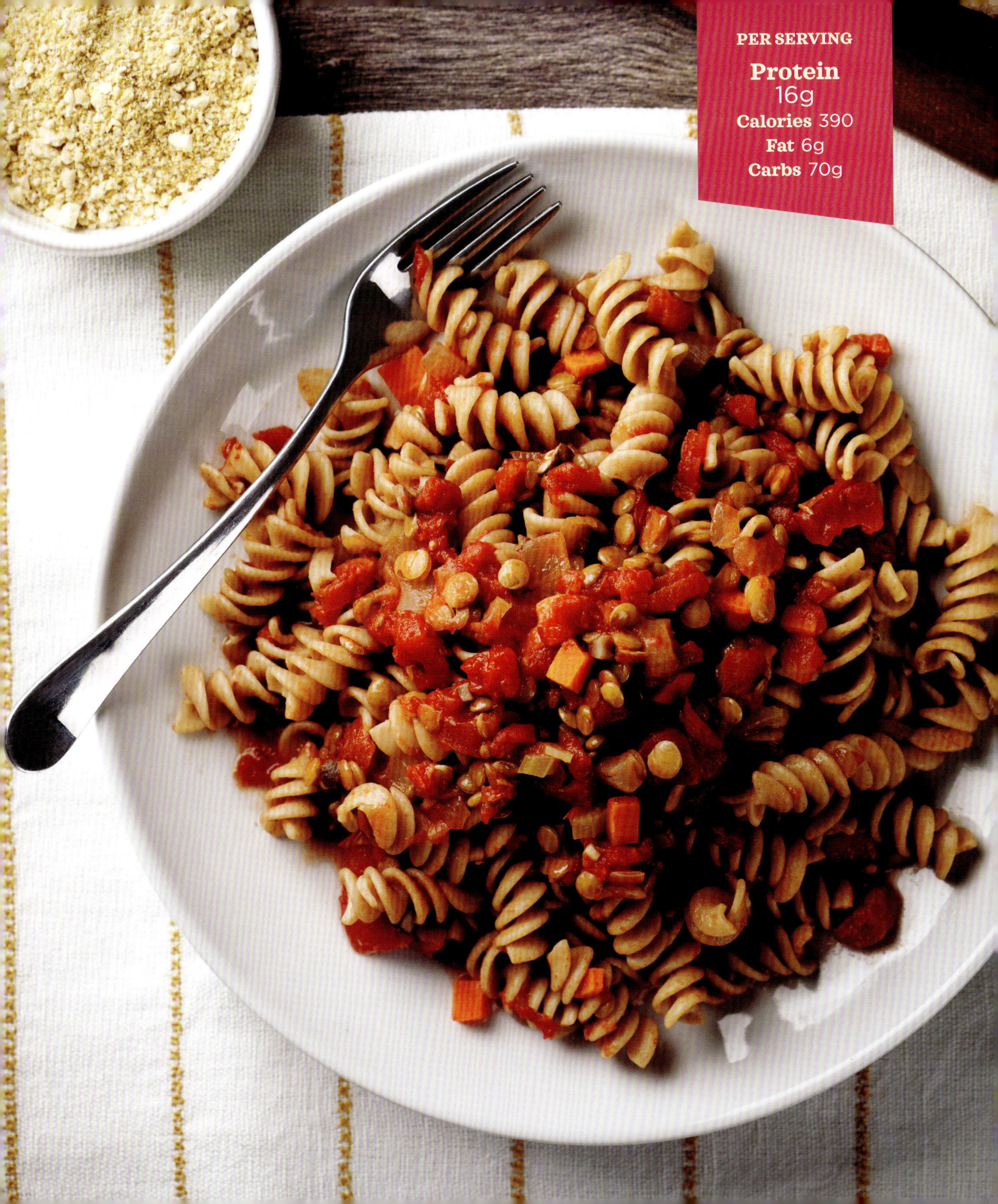
PER SERVING
Protein
16g
Calories 390
Fat 6g
Carbs 70g

Curried Beans and Greens

MAKES 6 SERVINGS

- **1 cup dried adzuki beans* or light red kidney beans**
- **4 cups plus 2 tablespoons cold water, plus additional for soaking**
- **2 pounds Swiss chard or kale**
- **1 tablespoon olive oil**
- **½ cup diced white onion**
- **2 cloves garlic, minced**
- **2 teaspoons sweet or spicy curry powder**
- **¼ teaspoon salt**
- **¼ teaspoon black pepper**

Adzuki beans are small reddish beans with a sweet flavor and high protein content. They are used in Japanese cooking and can be found at natural food markets.

1 Soak beans overnight in enough water to cover by at least 2 inches. Drain beans; rinse well.

2 Combine beans and 4 cups water in large saucepan; bring to a boil over high heat. Reduce heat to low; simmer 1 hour or until beans are tender. Drain beans.

3 Meanwhile, remove stems and ribs from greens; tear into large pieces.

4 Heat oil in large deep skillet over medium heat. Add onion and garlic; cook and stir 5 minutes or until onion is soft and translucent. Add curry powder; cook and stir 30 seconds or until slightly toasted and aromatic.

5 Add greens and remaining 2 tablespoons water to skillet; cook 5 minutes or until greens are wilted, stirring occasionally. Add beans; cook and stir until heated through. Season with salt and pepper.

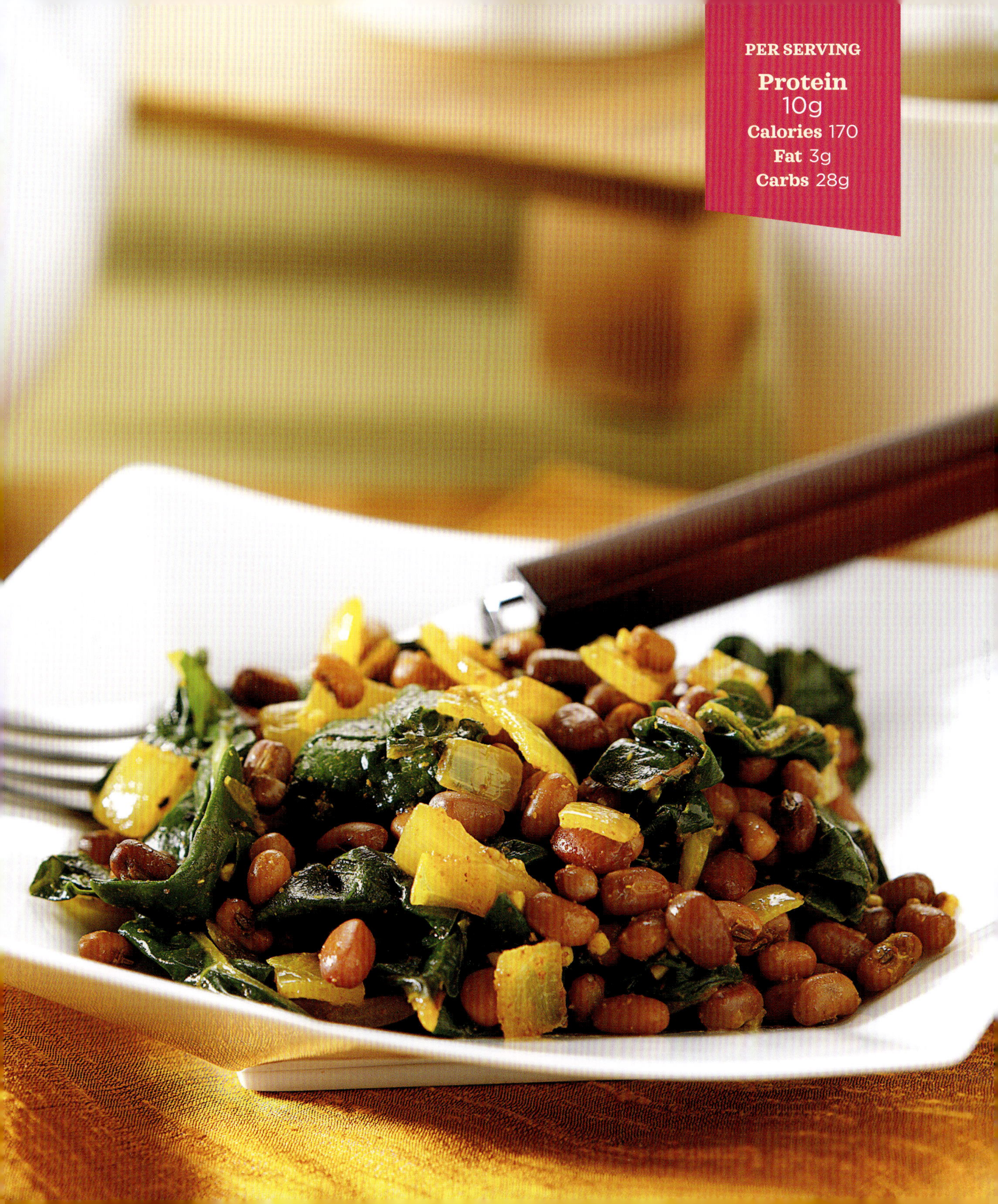
PER SERVING
Protein 10g
Calories 170
Fat 3g
Carbs 28g

Fresh Vegetable Lasagna

MAKES 8 SERVINGS

- 8 ounces uncooked lasagna noodles
- 1 package (10 ounces) frozen chopped spinach, thawed and squeezed dry
- 1 cup shredded carrots
- ½ cup sliced green onions
- ½ cup sliced red bell pepper (1-inch pieces)
- ¼ cup chopped fresh parsley
- ½ teaspoon black pepper
- 1½ cups low-fat (1%) cottage cheese
- ½ cup buttermilk
- ½ cup plain fat-free yogurt
- 2 egg whites
- 1 cup sliced mushrooms
- 1 can (14 ounces) artichoke hearts, rinsed, drained and chopped
- 2 cups (8 ounces) shredded part-skim mozzarella cheese
- ¼ cup grated Parmesan cheese

1. Cook lasagna noodles according to package directions, omitting salt. Drain and rinse under cold water to stop cooking; drain and set aside.

2. Preheat oven to 375°F. Spray 13×9-inch baking pan with nonstick cooking spray.

3. Combine spinach, carrots, green onions, bell pepper, parsley and black pepper in large bowl; mix well. Combine cottage cheese, buttermilk, yogurt and egg whites in food processor or blender; process until smooth.

4. Arrange one third of lasagna noodles in bottom of prepared pan. Spread with half of cottage cheese mixture, half of vegetable mixture, half of mushrooms, half of artichokes and ¾ cup mozzarella. Repeat layers. Top with remaining noodles; sprinkle with remaining ½ cup mozzarella and Parmesan.

5. Cover and bake 30 minutes. Uncover; bake 20 minutes or until bubbly and heated through. Let stand 10 minutes before serving.

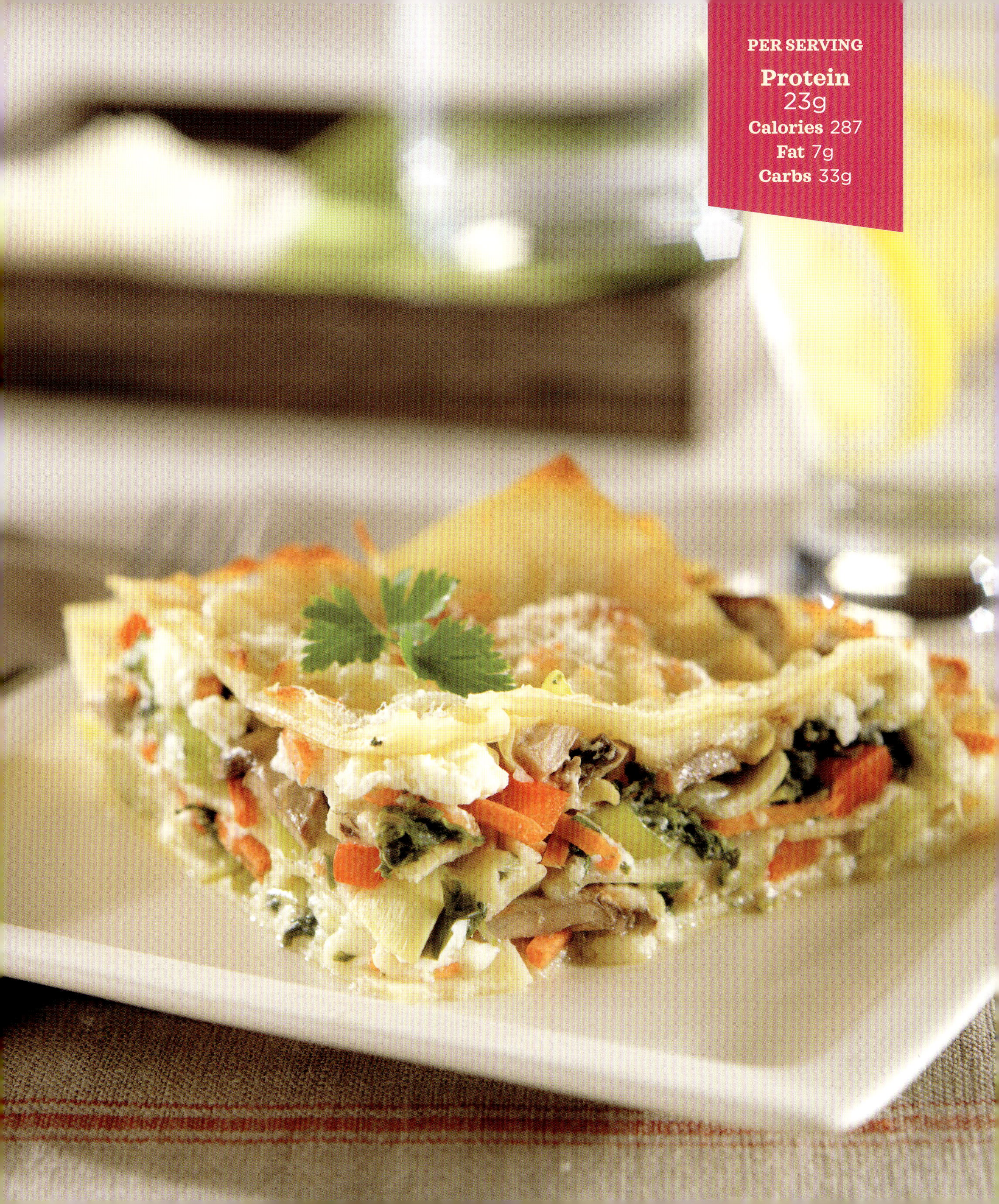
PER SERVING
Protein
23g
Calories 287
Fat 7g
Carbs 33g

PER SERVING
Protein
13g
Calories 340
Fat 9g
Carbs 54g

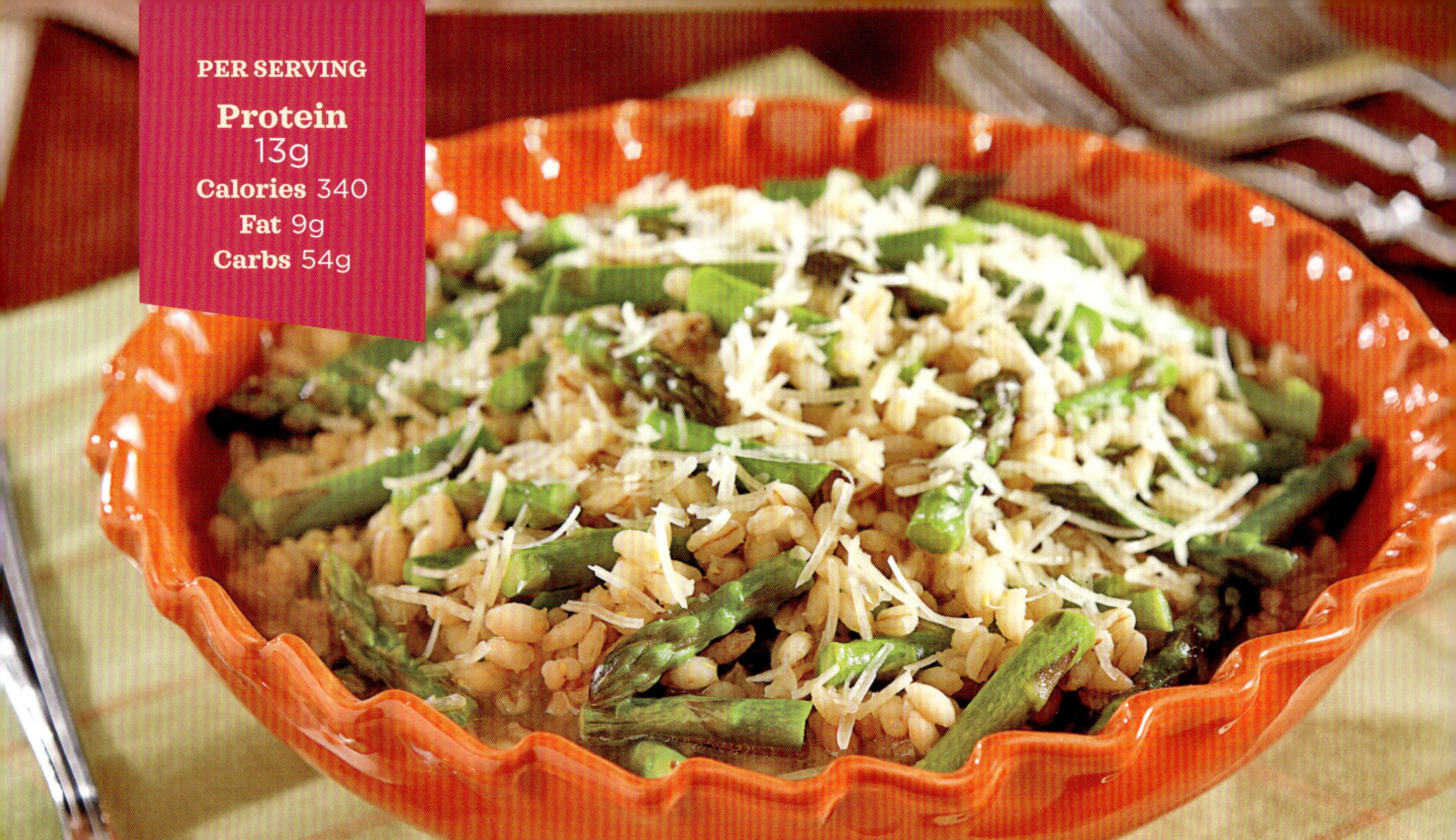

Asparagus Barley Risotto

MAKES 4 SERVINGS

- **2 tablespoons olive oil**
- **1 cup chopped onion**
- **1 clove garlic, minced**
- **1 teaspoon salt**
- **¼ teaspoon black pepper**
- **⅛ teaspoon dried marjoram**
- **1 cup uncooked pearl barley**
- **¼ cup dry white wine**
- **3 cups vegetable broth**
- **2 cups cut asparagus (1-inch pieces)**
- **¼ cup shredded Parmesan cheese**

1. Heat oil in medium saucepan over medium heat. Add onion; cook and stir 5 minutes or until softened. Add garlic, salt, pepper and marjoram; cook and stir 1 minute. Add barley; cook and stir 3 minutes or until toasted. Add wine; cook and stir 1 minute or until wine is absorbed.

2. Stir in broth; bring to a boil. Reduce heat to low; cover and simmer 20 minutes or until barley is tender, stirring occasionally.

3. Stir in asparagus; cover and cook until asparagus is tender and liquid has evaporated. Sprinkle with cheese just before serving.

PER SERVING
Protein
15g
Calories 125
Fat 1g
Carbs 13g

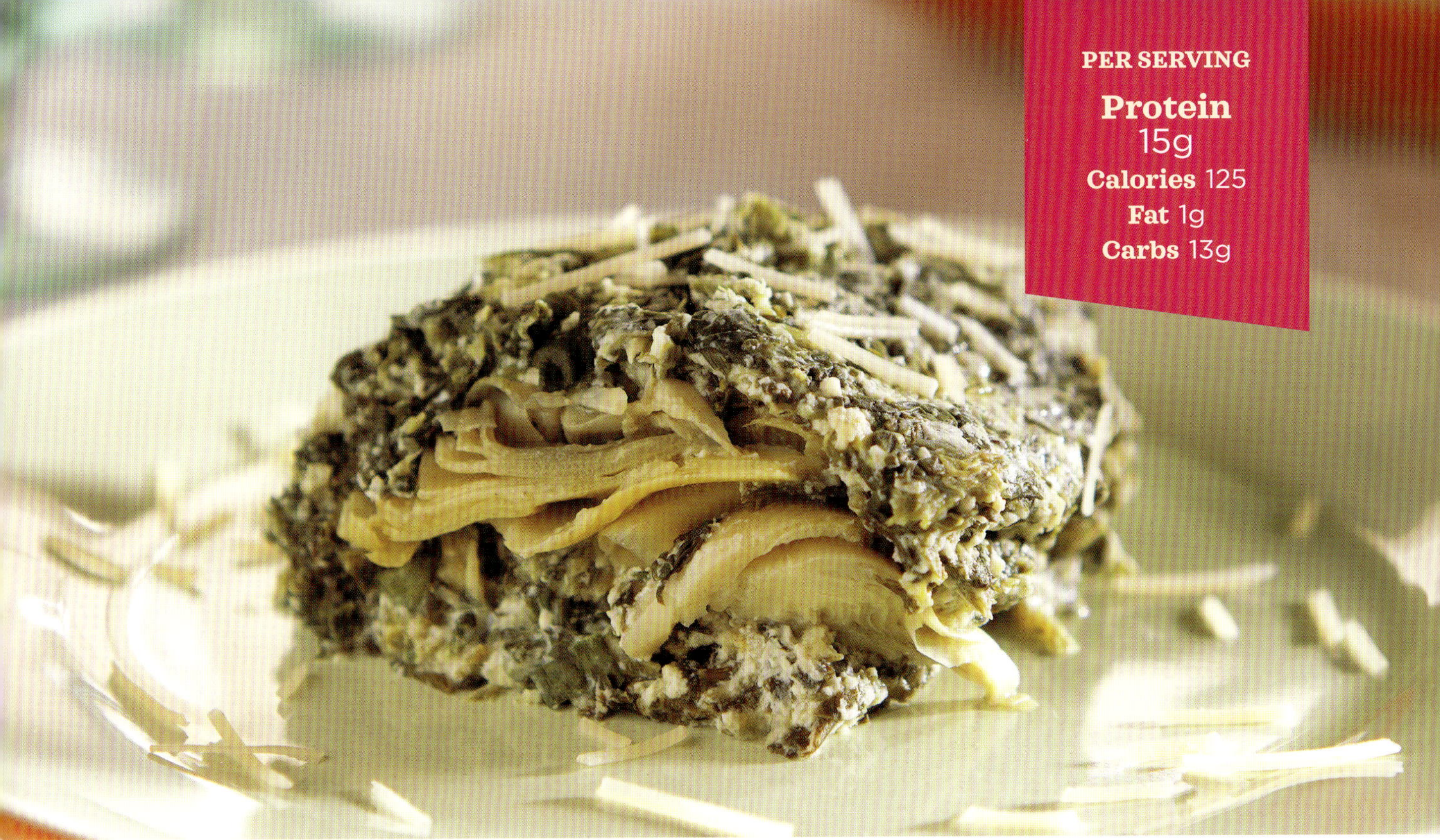

Spinach Artichoke Gratin

MAKES 6 SERVINGS

- 2 cups fat-free cottage cheese
- ½ cup liquid egg substitute
- 4½ tablespoons grated Parmesan cheese, divided
- 1 tablespoon lemon juice
- ⅛ teaspoon black pepper
- ⅛ teaspoon ground nutmeg
- 2 packages (10 ounces each) frozen chopped spinach, thawed
- ⅓ cup thinly sliced green onions
- 1 package (10 ounces) frozen artichoke hearts, thawed and halved

1. Preheat oven to 375°F. Spray 1½-quart baking dish with nonstick cooking spray.
2. Combine cottage cheese, egg substitute, 3 tablespoons Parmesan, lemon juice, pepper and nutmeg in food processor or blender; process until smooth.
3. Squeeze moisture from spinach. Combine spinach, cottage cheese mixture and green onions in large bowl; mix well. Spread half of mixture in prepared baking dish.
4. Pat artichokes dry with paper towels; place in single layer over spinach mixture. Sprinkle with remaining 1½ tablespoons Parmesan; top with remaining spinach mixture.
5. Cover and bake 25 minutes.

Curry Red Lentil and Chickpea Stew

MAKES 6 SERVINGS

- 1 tablespoon olive oil
- 1 onion, chopped
- 3 cloves garlic, minced
- 2 tablespoons minced fresh ginger
- 1 tablespoon curry powder
- 2 teaspoons ground turmeric
- 1 teaspoon salt
- ⅛ teaspoon ground red pepper
- 1 container (32 ounces) vegetable broth
- 1¼ cups dried red lentils
- 1 can (about 15 ounces) chickpeas, rinsed and drained
- 1 can (14 ounces) coconut milk
- 1 package (about 5 ounces) baby spinach

1. Heat oil in large saucepan over medium-high heat. Add onion; cook and stir 5 minutes or until softened. Add garlic, ginger, curry powder, turmeric, salt and red pepper; cook and stir 1 minute.
2. Stir in broth; bring to a boil. Stir in lentils; cook 15 minutes.
3. Stir in chickpeas and coconut milk; cook 5 to 10 minutes or until lentils are tender, chickpeas are heated through and stew is slightly thickened.
4. Stir in spinach; cook and stir 2 to 3 minutes or just until spinach is wilted. Taste and season with additional salt, if desired.

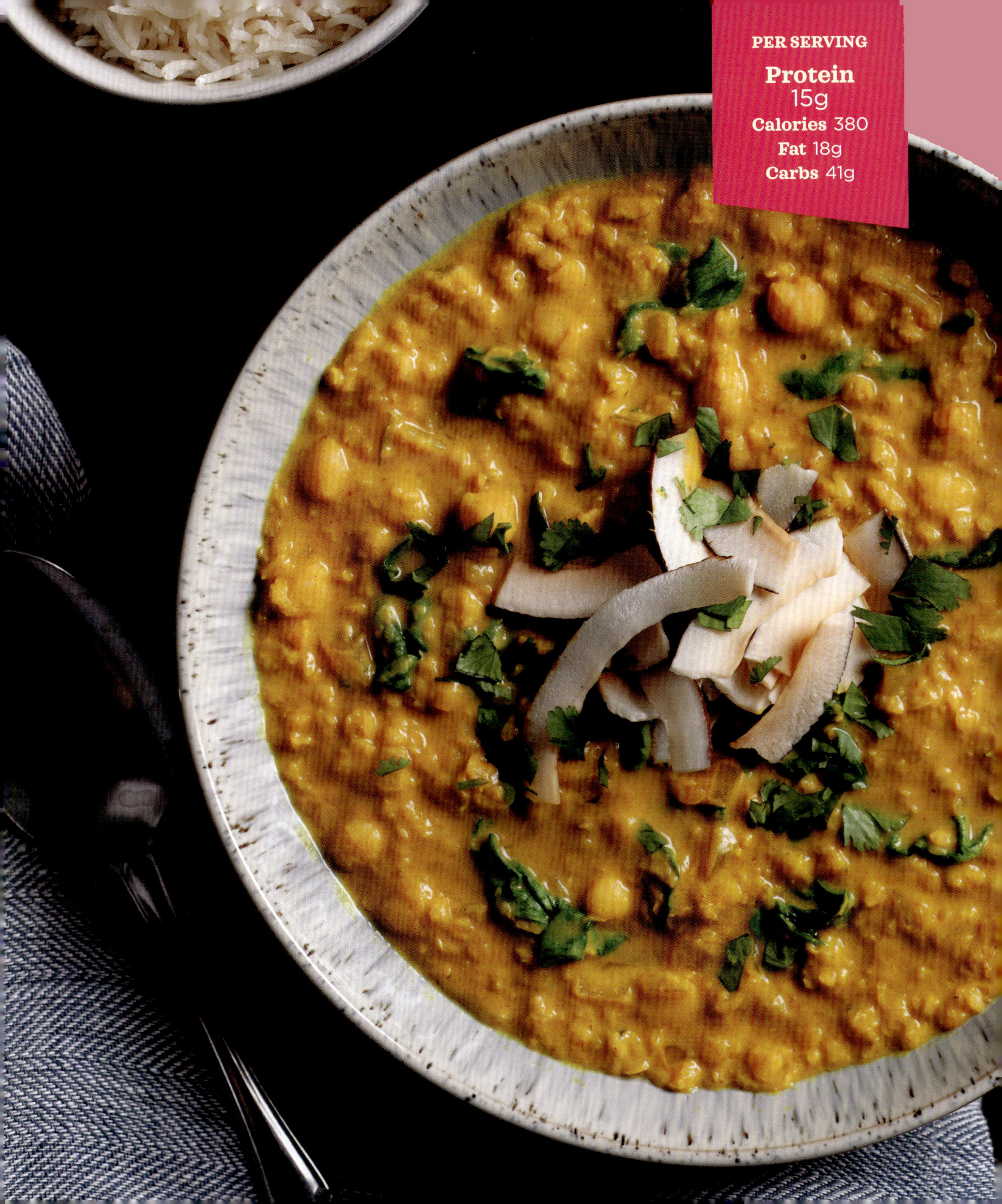
PER SERVING
Protein
15g
Calories 380
Fat 18g
Carbs 41g

Greek White Bean Risotto

MAKES 5 SERVINGS

- **3 teaspoons vegetarian chicken-flavor bouillon granules**
- **3 cloves garlic, minced**
- **1½ cups uncooked arborio rice**
- **2 teaspoons dried oregano leaves**
- **⅓ cup finely chopped sun-dried tomatoes (not packed in oil)**
- **1 cup canned cannellini beans, rinsed and drained**
- **¾ cup (3 ounces) crumbled feta cheese**
- **⅓ cup grated Parmesan cheese**
- **1 teaspoon lemon juice**
- **½ teaspoon black pepper**

1. Combine 5½ cups water and bouillon granules in large saucepan; bring to a simmer over medium-low heat.

2. Spray large saucepan with cooking spray; heat over medium heat. Add garlic; cook and stir 1 minute. Add rice and oregano; cook and stir 1 minute. Reduce heat to medium-low.

3. Add 1 cup hot broth; cook until broth is absorbed, stirring constantly. Add ½ cup hot broth; cook until broth is absorbed, stirring constantly. Stir in sun-dried tomatoes.

4. Add remaining hot broth, ½ cup at a time, stirring constantly until broth is absorbed before adding next ½ cup. (Total cooking time is about 35 minutes or until rice is tender but still firm to the bite.)

5. Add beans; cook and stir 1 minute. Remove from heat; stir in feta, Parmesan, lemon juice and pepper. Cover and let stand 5 minutes, stirring once. Garnish as desired.

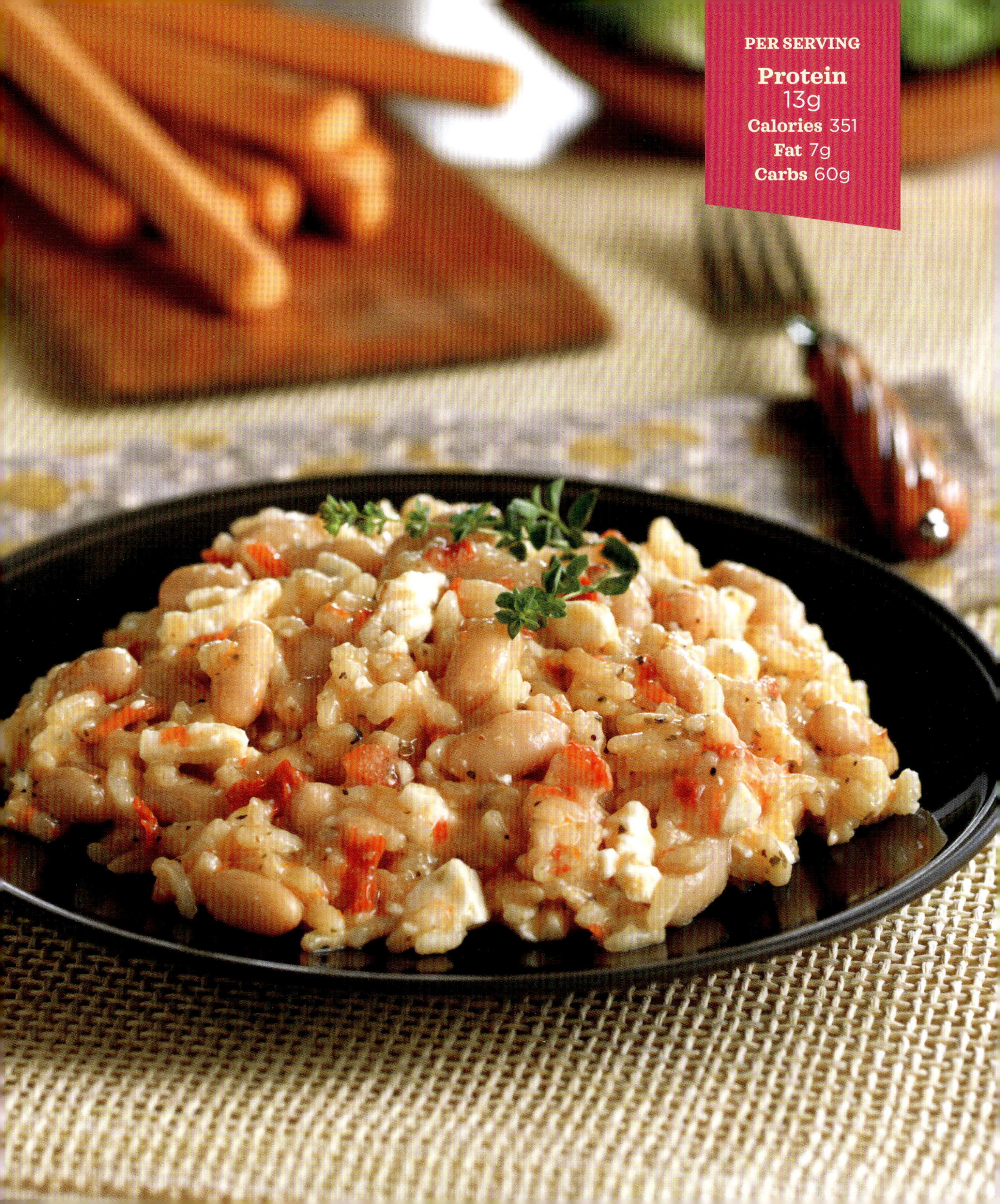
PER SERVING
Protein
13g
Calories 351
Fat 7g
Carbs 60g

Brown Rice with Chickpeas, Spinach and Feta

MAKES 4 SERVINGS

- ½ cup diced celery
- 2 cups water
- 1 can (about 15 ounces) reduced-sodium chickpeas, rinsed and drained
- 1 package (10 ounces) frozen chopped spinach, thawed and squeezed dry
- ½ cup uncooked instant brown rice
- 1 teaspoon Greek or Italian seasoning
- 1 clove garlic, minced
- ¼ teaspoon salt (optional)
- ⅛ teaspoon black pepper
- ½ cup (2 ounces) crumbled reduced-fat feta cheese
- 1 tablespoon lemon juice

1. Spray large skillet with nonstick cooking spray; heat over medium-high heat. Add celery; cook 4 minutes or until lightly browned in spots, stirring occasionally.

2. Stir in water, chickpeas, spinach, rice, Greek seasoning, garlic, salt, if desired, and pepper; bring to a boil. Reduce heat to low; cover and simmer 12 minutes or until rice is tender.

3. Remove from heat; stir in cheese and lemon juice.

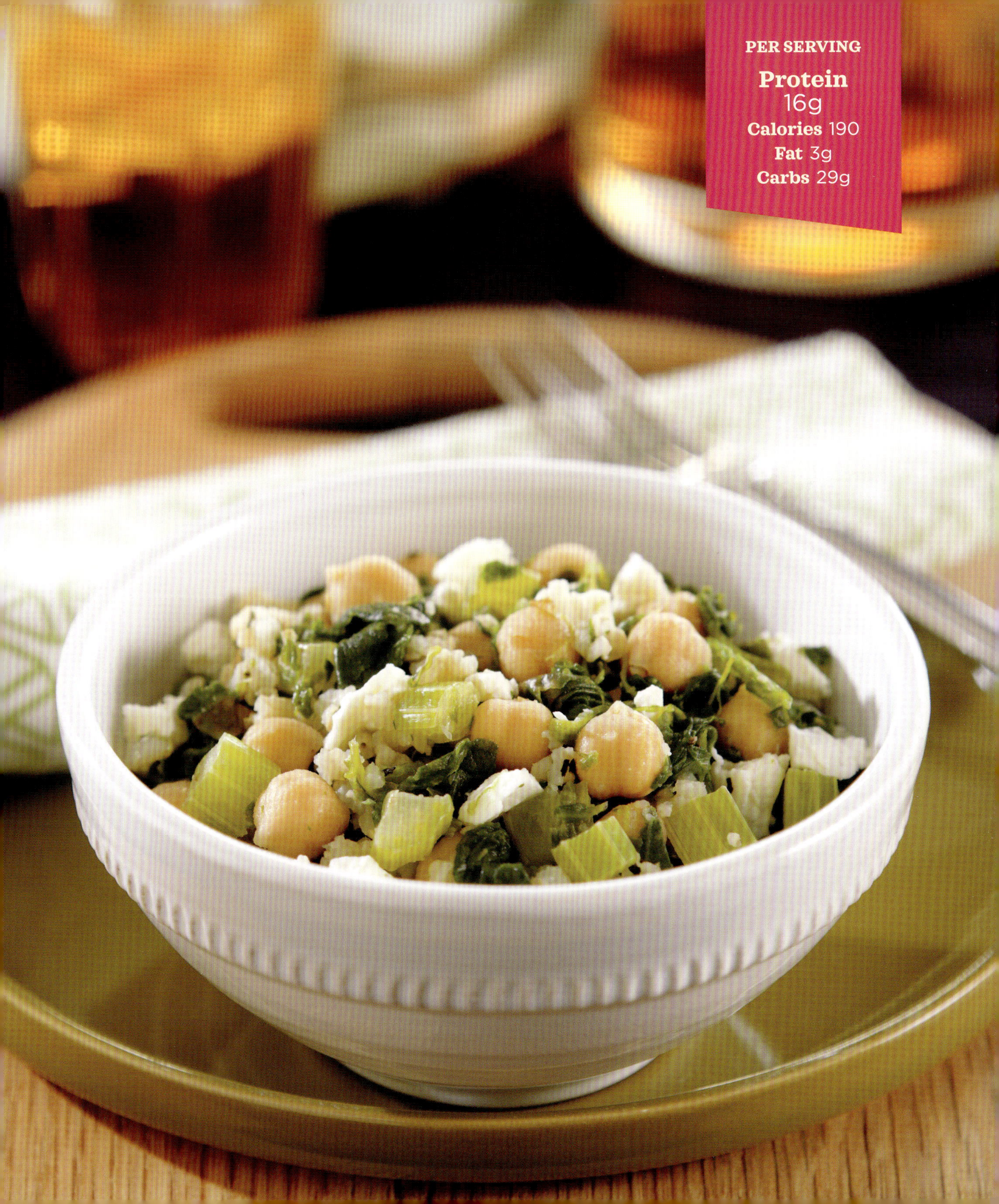
PER SERVING
Protein
16g
Calories 190
Fat 3g
Carbs 29g

PER SERVING
Protein
18g
Calories 310
Fat 8g
Carbs 45g

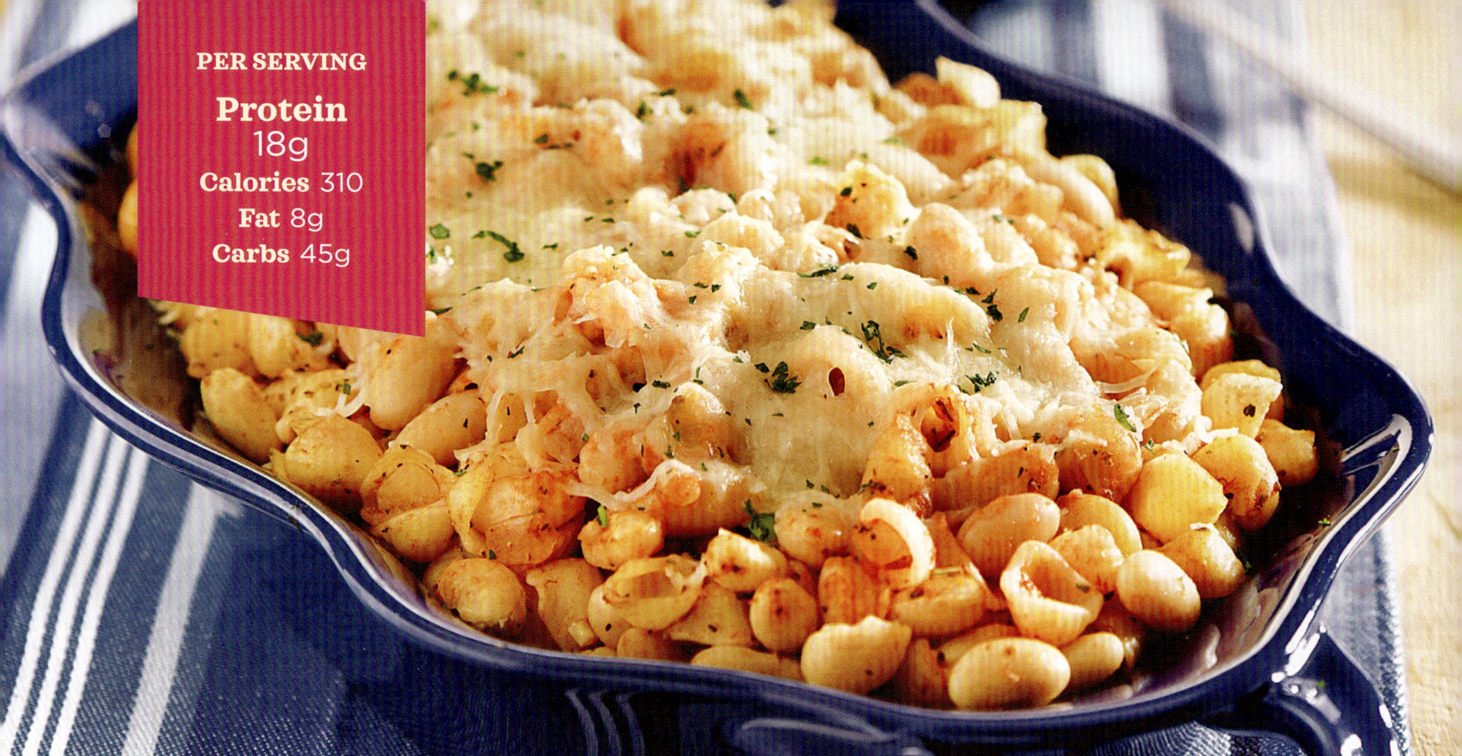

Pasta and White Bean Casserole

MAKES 6 SERVINGS

- 1 tablespoon olive oil
- ½ cup chopped onion
- 2 cloves garlic, minced
- 2 cans (about 15 ounces each) cannellini beans, rinsed and drained
- 3 cups cooked small shell pasta
- 1 can (8 ounces) tomato sauce
- 1½ teaspoons Italian seasoning
- ½ teaspoon salt
- ½ teaspoon black pepper
- 1 cup (4 ounces) shredded Italian cheese blend
- 2 tablespoons finely chopped fresh Italian parsley

1. Preheat oven to 350°F. Spray 2-quart baking dish with nonstick cooking spray.

2. Heat oil in large skillet over medium-high heat. Add onion and garlic; cook and stir 3 minutes or until onion is tender.

3. Add beans, pasta, tomato sauce, Italian seasoning, salt and pepper; mix well. Spoon into prepared baking dish; sprinkle with cheese and parsley.

4. Bake 20 minutes or until cheese is melted.

PER SERVING
Protein
13g
Calories 260
Fat 7g
Carbs 39g

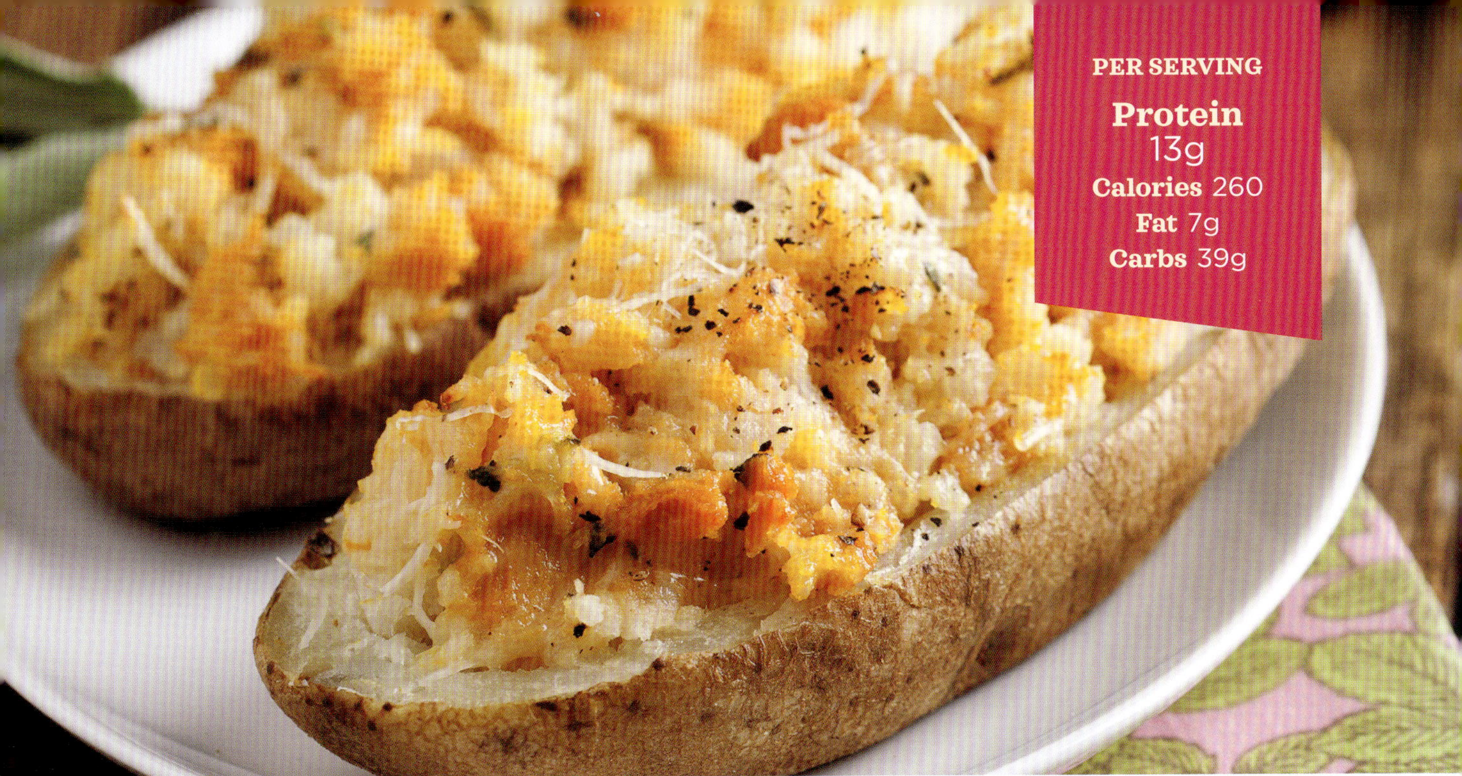

Pumpkin Parmesan Twice-Baked Potatoes

MAKES 4 SERVINGS

- **2 baking potatoes (about 12 ounces each)**
- **1 cup shredded Parmesan cheese**
- **6 tablespoons half-and-half**
- **¼ cup canned pumpkin**
- **1½ teaspoons minced fresh sage *or* ¼ teaspoon dried thyme**
- **¼ teaspoon salt**
- **⅛ teaspoon black pepper**

1. Preheat oven to 400°F. Scrub potatoes; pierce in several places with fork or small knife. Place potatoes directly on oven rack; bake 1 hour or until soft.

2. When cool enough to handle, cut potatoes in half lengthwise. Scoop out most of potato pulp into medium bowl, leaving thin potato shell. Mash potatoes with fork. Add cheese, half-and-half, pumpkin, sage, salt and pepper; mix well.

3. Place potato shells on baking sheet; spoon pumpkin mixture into shells. Bake 10 minutes or until filling is heated through.

Southwestern Lentil Burgers

MAKES 4 SERVINGS

- 2 cups water
- ¾ cup dried green lentils, rinsed and sorted
- 2 cloves garlic, minced
- 1 teaspoon chili powder
- 1 teaspoon ground cumin
- ⅛ teaspoon ground red pepper
- 3 egg whites
- ⅓ cup plain dry bread crumbs
- ¼ cup finely chopped fresh cilantro or green onions
- 2 teaspoons canola oil
- 4 whole wheat low-carb hamburger buns, split and lightly toasted
- ⅓ cup salsa
- ½ ripe avocado, sliced

1. Combine water and lentils in medium saucepan; bring to a boil over high heat. Reduce heat to medium-low; cover and simmer 20 minutes or until lentils are tender. Drain well. (Do not rinse.)

2. With motor running, drop garlic cloves through feed tube of food processor; process until minced. Add 1¼ cups lentils, chili powder, cumin and red pepper; process until lentils are minced.

3. Place remaining lentils in large bowl. Add egg whites, bread crumbs, cilantro and minced lentil mixture; mix well.

4. Shape mixture into four patties about 4 inches in diameter. Place on plate; cover and refrigerate at least 30 minutes or up to 2 hours.

5. Heat oil in large nonstick skillet over medium heat. Add patties; cook 5 minutes per side or until golden brown. Serve on buns topped with salsa and avocado.

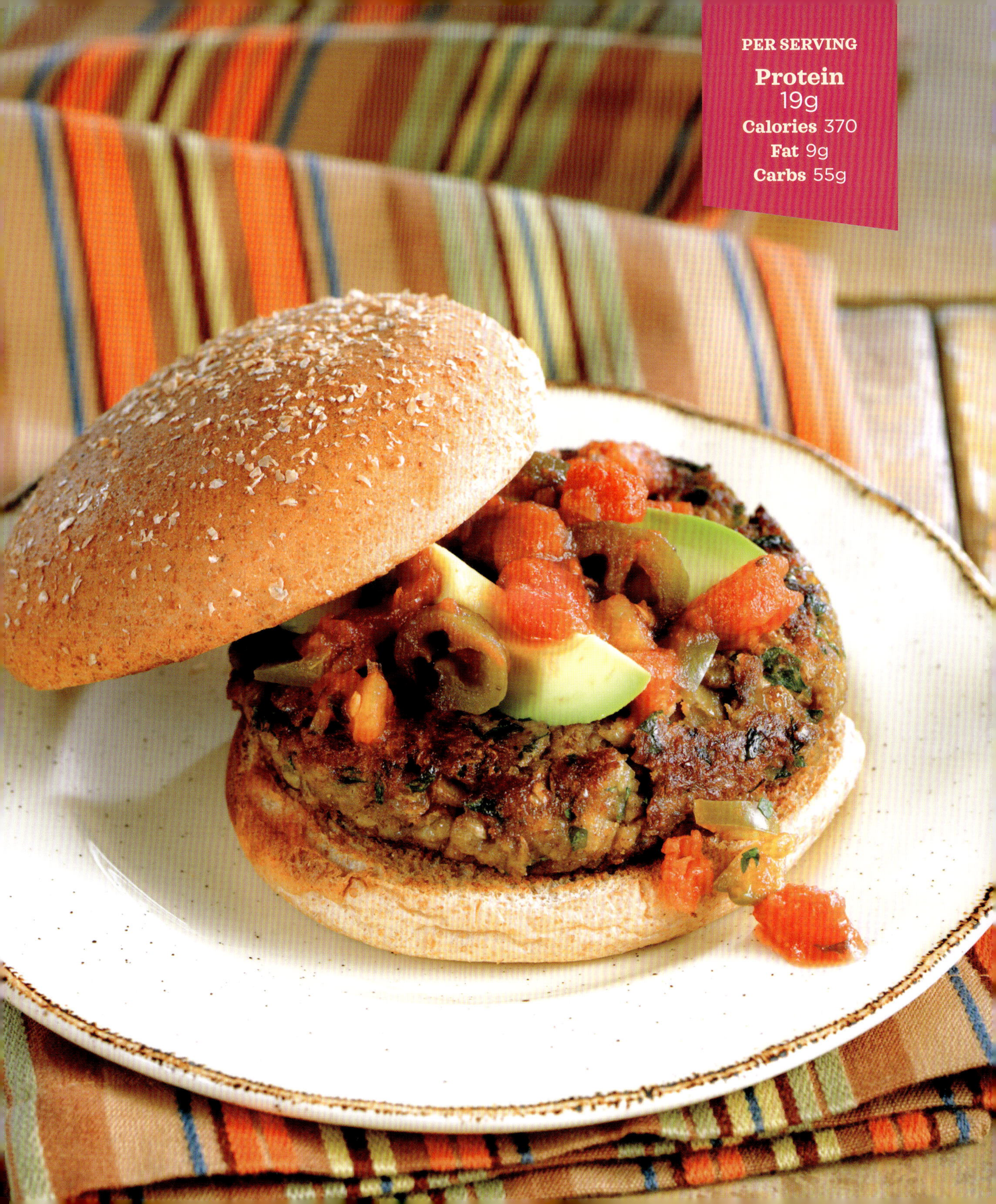
PER SERVING
Protein
19g
Calories 370
Fat 9g
Carbs 55g

D

E

F

G

H

I

K

L

M

N

O

P

Q

R

S

METRIC CONVERSION CHART

VOLUME MEASUREMENTS (dry)

1/8 teaspoon = 0.5 mL
1/4 teaspoon = 1 mL
1/2 teaspoon = 2 mL
3/4 teaspoon = 4 mL
1 teaspoon = 5 mL
1 tablespoon = 15 mL
2 tablespoons = 30 mL
1/4 cup = 60 mL
1/3 cup = 75 mL
1/2 cup = 125 mL
2/3 cup = 150 mL
3/4 cup = 175 mL
1 cup = 250 mL
2 cups = 1 pint = 500 mL
3 cups = 750 mL
4 cups = 1 quart = 1 L

VOLUME MEASUREMENTS (fluid)

1 fluid ounce (2 tablespoons) = 30 mL
4 fluid ounces (1/2 cup) = 125 mL
8 fluid ounces (1 cup) = 250 mL
12 fluid ounces (1 1/2 cups) = 375 mL
16 fluid ounces (2 cups) = 500 mL

WEIGHTS (mass)

1/2 ounce = 15 g
1 ounce = 30 g
3 ounces = 90 g
4 ounces = 120 g
8 ounces = 225 g
10 ounces = 285 g
12 ounces = 360 g
16 ounces = 1 pound = 450 g

DIMENSIONS

1/16 inch = 2 mm
1/8 inch = 3 mm
1/4 inch = 6 mm
1/2 inch = 1.5 cm
3/4 inch = 2 cm
1 inch = 2.5 cm

OVEN TEMPERATURES

250°F = 120°C
275°F = 140°C
300°F = 150°C
325°F = 160°C
350°F = 180°C
375°F = 190°C
400°F = 200°C
425°F = 220°C
450°F = 230°C

BAKING PAN SIZES

Utensil	Size in Inches/Quarts	Metric Volume	Size in Centimeters
Baking or Cake Pan (square or rectangular)	8×8×2	2 L	20×20×5
	9×9×2	2.5 L	23×23×5
	12×8×2	3 L	30×20×5
	13×9×2	3.5 L	33×23×5
Loaf Pan	8×4×3	1.5 L	20×10×7
	9×5×3	2 L	23×13×7
Round Layer Cake Pan	8×1½	1.2 L	20×4
	9×1½	1.5 L	23×4
Pie Plate	8×1¼	750 mL	20×3
	9×1¼	1 L	23×3
Baking Dish or Casserole	1 quart	1 L	—
	1½ quart	1.5 L	—
	2 quart	2 L	—